Sally Edwards'
Heart Zone
TRAINING

Sally Edwards'
Heart Zone
TRAINING

Exercise Smart, Stay Fit, and Live Longer

SALLY EDWARDS

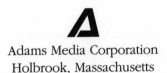

Adams Media Corporation
Holbrook, Massachusetts

Published by Adams Media Corporation
260 Center Street, Holbrook, MA 02343

ISBN: 1-55850-552-0

Printed in Canada

J I H G F

Library of Congress Cataloging-in-Publication Data
Edwards, Sally.
[Heart zone training]
Sally Edward's heart zone training : exercise smart, stay fit, and live longer / Sally Edwards.
p.   cm.
Includes index.
ISBN 1-55850-552-0 (pb)
1. Exercise. 2. Heart rate monitoring. 3. Physical fitness. I. Title.
RA781.E326   1996
613.7'1—dc20   96–19659
CIP

This publication is designed to provide accurate and authoritative information with regard to the subject matter covered. It is sold with the understanding that the publisher is not engaged in rendering legal, accounting, or other professional advice. If legal advice or other expert assistance is required, the services of a competent professional person should be sought.
— From a *Declaration of Principles* jointly adopted by a Committee of the American Bar Association and a Committee of Publishers and Associations

The questionnaire on page 19 has been adapted from the PAR-Q Physical Readiness Questionnaire developed by the British Columbia Ministry of Health. The questionnaire on pages 52–53 has been adapted from one prepared by the U.S. National Heart, Lung, and Blood Institute (1981). The table on page 58 has been adapted from one prepared by the Michigan Heart Association.

This book is available at quantity discounts for bulk purchases.
For information, call 1-800-872-5627 (in Massachusetts, 781-767-8100).

Visit our home page: www.adamsmedia.com

To each and every one of you who has struggled with exercise and diet programs and is willing to try one more time with a program that works for a lifetime. The integration of the mind, the body, and the spirit is what works in the long run, and that's what this book is all about.

Contents

Foreword

We're proud to know and work with Sally Edwards. An extraordinary professional athlete, she's always impressed us by keeping her sights on what can help ordinary women and men attain their health and fitness goals. Unlike many super-athletes, she doesn't put herself above or beyond the rest of us; she does the rough job of breaking trail so that the rest of us can follow her lead. We've long considered her a valuable ally to our fight for fitness, and we have no doubt that you will too.

Heart Zone Training, Sally Edwards's ninth book, stands out from many in the health and fitness field thanks to its keen understanding of, and sympathy for, the novice. However, every exerciser, of any level of skill and training, will gain insight into his or her efforts by reading it. Edwards's explanation of the levels of exercise and their uses are a must-read for both the beginner and the well-seasoned athlete.

This book is impressive—clear, accurate, and right on target—and the system *works*. We defy you to try the Heart Zone Training program and *not* get fit! Good luck to you, and congratulations on starting your new healthy lifestyle!

Covert Bailey and Lea Bishop
Authors of:
  Smart Exercise
  The New Fit or Fat
  The Fit or Fat Woman

Acknowledgments

Everyone who shared in this experience as an editor, supporter, counselor, athlete, or partner has earned a place on this page. I couldn't have done this without you.

Michael Snell put together the deal as the agent and then word-smithed it into perfection. Pat Snell tested the program by reading the manuscript and becoming an avid zone trainer. Ed Walters and the entire team at Adams Media Corporation took a manuscript and made it into what you are holding in your hands. Ellen Sampson, my sidekick, editor, friend, and training and business partner, came through when I needed help, as she has always done. Donna Lee did the early work on the manuscript as a labor of love. Jazz Spinnler Scheingraber edited the very rough drafts of the manuscript and added her competitive cross-country skier's perspective. Tracy Kelly did the mechanical and computer input stuff that only she loves. Ronda Gates became my business partner in Heart Lifestyles and supported me through those long hours as the book unfolded. She is my inspiration, business partner, and supporter. Randy Saks traveled with me for a year as we taught the material, and answered thousands of questions. He challenged, taught, showed, and lead me towards achieving our mission and movement—that of getting people fit. Amy Nelson was there in the early days as all of this unfolded. She introduced me to the aerobics industry, and we developed Heart Group Exercise and Heart Aerobics from her efforts. Linda Shelton came in at the last minute to challenge and push the concepts, the zones, and the training tree. Judy Stansbury took this material, developed it, and turned it into a high school physical education curriculum that is getting kids excited about exercise again. Linda Warren listened to a lecture and developed the Heart Walking program as a result. Helen Kahn gave me the insider's viewpoint of the typical reader of the book. Annie Bellman provided the comforts and conveniences that all authors need in her retreat home in Black Butte, Oregon.

Introduction
Let's Do It!

I hate long-winded introductions, and I hate sitting around reading about fitness when I could be doing something to keep fit. So let's get to know each other and start doing something together right off the bat.

I'm Sally Edwards and I wrote this book to change your life. I've been interested in health and fitness all my life, from studying exercise physiology in grad school to my volunteer service with the Red Cross in the Vietnam War to my various personal achievements in professional athletic competition. The longer I live, the surer I am that fitness is the key to not only health but happiness. Now, at age forty-eight, I have reached the inescapable, tried-and-true conclusion that Heart Zone Training is the best approach to all-around fitness I've ever seen.

Heart Zone Training starts with the premise that each of us is an individual. Because we are individuals, no single fitness regimen will give us all the same results. Fad diets and fad exercise programs exist to sell one idea, one plan, one routine to everybody, so it's not surprising that most people don't usually see the promised amazing results. The beauty of Heart Zone Training is that it respects you as an individual. Your body's feedback is what determines your personal fitness plan.

I bring to Heart Zone Training one more premise, that true fitness is fitness for life. Fitness needs to be a way of life to provide lasting results. People are often sold short by the promises of fads. Yes, such-and-such thirty-day program may take off ten pounds, but does it work in the long term? Is eating only celery and doing a hundred sit-ups a day the way you want to spend your life? For you, for me, for anyone to achieve lasting fitness, we have to have a program that makes sense with our lifestyles and is an efficient use of our exercise time. That's Heart Zone Training.

Who are you? You're the twenty-seven-year-old working mom who has decided the time is right to lose some weight (as long as you can find the time). You're a forty-two-year-old weekend runner who wants to move on to the next level of conditioning by getting more out of each workout. You're the sixty-one-year-old whose family has a history of heart problems. Regardless of your age, sex, weight, or present level of fitness, you share at least one goal with everyone else for whom I've written this book: You want to live a long, healthy, happy life.

I promised before that we would start doing something together right away, so we won't delay any further: Let's measure our heart rates.

Monitoring Your Heart Rate

There are two basic methods of measuring anyone's heart rate: manually (with your hands) or mechanically (with some sort of a heart rate monitor). If you want to take your heart rate manually, you should remember that your heart rate and your pulse rate are usually, but not necessarily, equal. "Heart rate" refers to the electrical impulses that cause your heart to beat, but "pulse rate" refers only to the movement of blood through your arteries.

Start by measuring your heart rate while sitting still. To measure your pulse manually, take two fingers, place them over the inside surface of your wrist, and lightly apply pressure. Wait quietly and move your fingers until you feel the blood flow. The pulse is taken in the wrist because it is safe and easy; taking your pulse rate from your neck's carotid artery can slow your heart rate and sometimes gives you a false reading. The easiest method is to count the number of pulse waves during 6 seconds and add a 0 to that number to obtain the number of beats per minute. If you count 7 beats in 6 seconds, then add a 0, you have the number 70, or 70 beats per minute.

Thanks to heart rate monitors, the mechanical method of heart rate measurement is a bit simpler. Now, when you think of heart rate monitors, you probably think of big machines in a doctor's office. Although it's true that there are plenty of multi-thousand-dollar pieces of electronic equipment out there that do a very nice job of measuring heart rate, that's not what I'm talking about. I'm a fan of the small, personal, accurate, and (relatively) inexpensive heart rate monitors that look a lot like wristwatches. You strap the receiver on your wrist and a thin, unobtrusive transmitter belt around your chest, and you're ready to go. Wearing a heart rate monitor keeps your hands free and gives you instant and continuous feedback.

However you measure your heart rate, jot down the number you get for one minute while at rest. It will probably be somewhere between 45 and 75. Having done that, pat yourself on the back, because you've just mastered the key to Heart Zone Training. For more details, meet me in Chapter 1!

Understanding Heart Zone Training

Welcome to the first day of your new life!

"Excuse me?" you say. "I'm just reading a book here. I'm not committing myself to some sort of life-changing, soul-searching Zonequest for personal transformation. I just want to get a little fitter, maybe lose those ten or twenty pounds that make me feel like I'm walking around with one of those lead vests the dentist makes you wear for x-rays. A 'new life'? Give me a break!"

Okay, so you may not have planned to embark on some big new phase of your life when you bought this book, but if you try just a little to practice the ideas I'll be sharing with you, then you WILL be starting a new life.

Do you know why you haven't been able to lose or keep off those extra pounds or to achieve or maintain the aerobic fitness that allows you climb three flights of stairs without panting? I do. It's because you haven't changed your life. You haven't chosen a fitness-based approach to living; you've just stuck a few out-of-date ideas on your mental refrigerator door, hoping they'd remind you to take a walk before treating yourself to a hot fudge sundae. That's not how long-term fitness works.

Think about your fit friends. Everybody knows one or two people who've made it to middle age or beyond in peak condition. They're trim, they're healthy, they play tennis, swim, walk, or bike their way through the week, and they look really good doing it. The passing years don't seem to have affected them. Why not? Well, at some point in their lives (maybe even as children, if they were lucky enough to have been born into a fit family), they chose a fitness-based lifestyle.

Once you do choose to make fitness the basis of your life, with time and patience it can become a snap to stay fit, but making the initial commitment can seem daunting. We've all got excuses: lack of time, not enough energy, boredom with an exercise routine, inconvenience, or that popular, "I'll do it tomorrow." Whatever your excuse, write it down and stick it on your real refrigerator door. This, and nothing else, is keeping you off the road to a fitter, healthier, happier life. Now you have something to do: Stop making that excuse. Replace "I'm too busy" with "I'm setting aside fifteen minutes, three days a week, to exercise." Instead of telling yourself, "I'm too tired," tell yourself, "Exercising gives me energy—it doesn't take it away." Rather than protesting that "Walking two miles bores me to death," remind yourself that "I can take this time to smell the roses along the way."

It all begins with commitment. Once you've made a commitment to fitness, you can begin using Heart Zone

Training immediately, whether you walk or run or play tennis or use a stationary bicycle. You don't have to work out in a gym, although that can be fun and motivating. You don't have to spend a lot of time; fifteen minutes, three times a week will do for starters. You don't have to be bursting with unused energy, although you may be after you start your new fitness-based life. You don't have to be fit already—but if you are, there's a lot Heart Zone Training can do for you, too.

The bottom line: If you seriously wish to achieve a life of fitness, Heart Zone Training will enable you to make that transformation gently and easily.

Welcome.

Work Your Body, Work Your Heart

"So," you say, "What is Heart Zone Training, and how can it change my life?"

Simply put, Heart Zone Training is a fitness program. It's a simple, sensible way to make the most of your workouts by monitoring the intensity of the efforts of the key muscle in your body: the heart. Throughout the book I'll be talking about how Heart Zone Training works. Little by little you'll get an exact picture of the mechanisms at work in making (and keeping) you fit.

To begin with, when you expend effort, whether by mowing the lawn, running up a hill, or swimming a few fast laps at the pool, you increase your body's workload. Increasing your effort, or workload, in turn increases your heart rate. We in the fitness profession call that degree of effort "intensity." I'm sure you've probably heard people talk about doing really "intense" workouts, when they wanted to push themselves, or "not very intense" workouts, when they didn't. The thing is, if you want to exercise efficiently, you've got to have a better way to measure your effort intensity than just "guesstimating." There is a way, and competitive athletes and other fitness professionals have been doing it for years to very good effect. We measure exercise intensity by measuring our heart rates.

Your heart is one big muscle, and it does its work by repeatedly expanding and contracting, drawing blood in and then pushing it out again, somewhat like the opening and closing of a fist. The number of times per minute that your heart muscle squeezes, or contracts, is your heart rate in beats per minute (bpm).

In the introduction you learned how to measure your heart rate manually by taking your pulse while sitting still and completely relaxed. The number you recorded was your *ambient heart rate.* Most people's ambient heart rate hovers around 70 bpm. You can also measure your heart rate when you first wake up in the morning (before you get out of bed) to find what is called your *resting heart rate.* Most people's resting heart rate is about 5 bpm lower than their ambient heart rate. As a rule of thumb, the lower these numbers are the better. The resting heart rates of world-class athletes can fall in the low thirties. This means that their heart beats once, waits two seconds, and then beats again. Their hearts don't have to contract very often because they've achieved cardiac efficiency: Their blood vessels are wide open, with no resistance from such obstacles as cholesterol buildup. That is why their heart doesn't have to beat as often as an unfit person's to move the same amount of blood. You may never compete in a marathon, but you want to achieve the same heart rate goals as the professional runner: low ambient and resting heart rate numbers.

When you stand up and start walking around, your heart rate goes up, because you are making your body, and therefore your heart, work a little harder. That's called *increased workload.* If you carry a twenty-five pound baby around, your heart rate will go up even further, because you have just increased the intensity of your effort. The higher the intensity, the higher the workload, the higher the heart rate.

So as you increase the intensity of your effort, your heart rate increases—say from 60 bpm while sitting in a recliner and watching the evening news to 120 bpm while walking briskly uphill to 180 bpm while sprinting for the finish line of a 5K run. Now, at different points along this progression from 60 bpm to 180 bpm, you pass into different heart zones. In the most basic sense, a heart rate zone is a range of heart beats per minute, say from 120 bpm to 140 bpm. We don't usually talk about these zones in fixed numbers, though. Usually heart rate zones are expressed as percentages of your maximum heart rate (Max HR).

The zones vary somewhat from person to person, depending upon one's Max HR, so to find your own zones you must determine what your maximum heart rate is. Max HR is the greatest number of contractions your heart can make in one minute. For example, if I run as fast and as hard as I can, which I can only do for less than a minute at full speed, my heart will beat progressively faster and faster and faster until it reaches a peak, or maximum number of beats per minute. My Max HR at the age of forty-eight, is 200 bpm. Now, what does this number really mean?

About Your Maximum Heart Rate

Finding out your maximum heart rate is the first step in Heart Zone Training. But before you do that, here are some important things to know:

- Max HR is genetically determined (you're born with it).
- Max HR is a relatively fixed number, unless you become unfit.
- Max HR cannot be increased by training.
- Max HR declines with age only in relatively sedentary individuals.
- Max HR is affected by drugs such as beta blockers.
- Max HR in the high range does not predict better athletic performance.
- Max HR in the low range does not predict poorer athletic performance.
- Max HR varies greatly among people of the same age.
- Max HR for children can be over 200 bpm.
- Max HR cannot be accurately predicted by any mathematic formula.
- Max HR testing requires the person to be fully rested.
- Max HR testing needs to be done several times to be accurate.

There's one more point to remember:

- Max HR provides the best number to use as an anchor point for an individual's training zones.

Max HR is a crucial piece of information, since you design your entire Heart Zone Training program around it. There are a number of different approaches to determining this number. These include taking a professionally administered Max HR test to determine the exact number or performing your own sub-maximum test, which will give you a fairly accurate number.

When you do this, remember that Max HR is activity-specific. You need to know your Max HR for each of the activities you may be zone training in. If you are going to set your zones as a cyclist, you need a biking Max HR test; if you're going to set them as a runner, you need a running Max HR test.

If you aren't in tip-top shape and haven't been for a while, you don't want to take a Max HR test designed to bring you to your actual Max HR. Instead you should rely on the less-intense best-guess methods. These methods, though not precise, will allow you to begin Heart Zone Training. They use sub-maximum (SubMax) testing to predict your Max HR. Though not perfect, these test/formula approaches give you more accurate data than mathematical formulas alone, because the results factor in actual numbers specific to you. **Remember, before you take these tests, you should consult your physician to make sure you can do so safely.**

First of all, pinpoint your current level of cardiovascular (not muscular) fitness:

CURRENT CONDITION

Poor Shape—You do not exercise at all, or you have not exercised recently (last eight weeks). Remember, you can be thin and outwardly healthy and still be in poor cardiovascular shape.

Average Shape—You walk a mile three times a week, or participate in any aerobic activity three times a week for twenty minutes.

Excellent Shape—You exercise regularly more than one hour a week, or you walk or run at least five miles a week.

With your fitness level in mind you can now administer one or both of the following SubMax tests. Before taking any test or working out, you should warm up by exercising gently for a few minutes.

TEST 1: The SubMax One-Mile Walking Test. Go to any high school or college track (most are 400 meters or 440 yards around) and walk or stride as fast as you can in your current condition. Don't use a "race-walking" technique—with huge arm swings and hip rotations—just your normal, comfortable walking style. Walk four continuous evenly paced and vigorous laps (one mile). The first three laps will put you on a heart rate plateau or steady state, where you will remain for the last lap. The last lap is the important one. Determine your average heart rate for only the last lap.

Add to this average last-lap heart rate the number that best matches your current fitness level. For SubMax Test 1, if you are in poor shape, add 40 bpm. If you are in average shape, add 50 bpm. If you are in excellent shape, add 60 bpm.

For example, a person in poor shape might have an average heart rate of 120 bpm for the last lap. Adding 40 bpm to that makes a Max HR of 160 bpm. Another person, in average shape, recorded 125 bpm for the last lap, then added 50 bpm for a total of 175. For myself, a person in excellent shape, I would add 60 bpm to my last lap's heart rate of 135 bpm, for a Max HR of 195, which is pretty close to my true Max HR of 200 bpm.

TEST 2: The SubMax Step Test. Use an eight-inch step (almost any step in your home or in an athletic club will do) and perform a three-minute step test. After your warm-up, step up and down in a four-count sequence as follows: right foot up, left up, right down, left down. Each time you move a foot up or down, it counts as one step. Count "Up, up, down, down" for one set, with twenty sets to the minute. It is very important that you don't speed up the pace. Keep it regular.

After two minutes you'll need to measure your heart rate during the last minute. You can now predict your Max HR by adding to your last minute's average heart rate one of the following numbers. For SubMax Test 2, if you are in poor shape, add 55 bpm. If you are in average shape, add 65 bpm. If you are in excellent shape, add 75 bpm.

For example, a person in poor shape might measure 130 bpm during the last minute of the test, then add 55 to come up with a Max HR of 185 bpm. Another person, in average shape, might have found their average heart rate to be 125 bpm; when they add 65, they find their Max HR to be about 190 bpm. For myself, as I'm in excellent shape, I'd add 75 to an average heart rate of 115 to find a Max HR of 190 bpm.

Understanding Heart Rate Zones

You may already have heard of the target heart rate zone. You may have seen wall charts at the gym or in a medical office that graphically display some sort of relationship between exercise heart rate and age. Those wall charts try to give you a target range of heart rates, usually a zone of 70 to 85 percent of the expected Max HR for your age and sex, within which you are supposed to exercise in order to gain the greatest benefit. Unfortunately, since heart rate zones depend more upon your Max HR than your age, these numbers can be misleading. The 70 percent floor and the 85 percent ceiling of the zone are too high and too hard for most people to exercise within. As a result, most people who have tried to work out within this zone have gotten discouraged and quit.

Remember this rule: No one heart rate zone applies to everyone. Seldom, in fact, does only one heart rate zone make sense for one individual. In time you will come to set several heart rate zones for yourself, each of which you can use to achieve different benefits. If you want to lose weight, for instance, you'll work out in a zone quite different from the one you would use to strengthen your heart, or the one that increases your overall endurance and athletic performance. That's the key to Heart Zone Training: You choose which benefit you want from exercise, then you tailor a program accordingly.

Heart Zone Training involves five zones, each of which has different fitness benefits.

THE FIVE HEART RATE ZONES

ZONE	% OF MAX HR	FOR 200 BPM MAX HR	BENEFIT	EXERCISE EXAMPLE
REDLINE	100-90%	200–180 bpm	Improves athletic performance	running all out
ANAEROBIC (THRESHOLD)	90–80%	180-160 bpm	Improves endurance	running very fast
AEROBIC	80-70%	160–140 bpm	Enhances cardiovascular strength	running easily
TEMPERATE	70-60%	140–120 bpm	Burns high percentage of fat	jogging easily
HEALTHY HEART	60–50%	120-100 bpm	Strengthens your heart	walking briskly

Your Healthy Heart zone is from 50 to 60 percent of your Max HR. This zone is ideal for beginners, because it's fun, it's comfortable, it creates cardiovascular benefits, it burns some fat, and gives you a clear sense of accomplishment. For me this zone is 100 to 120 bpm (50 percent to 60 percent of my

Max HR of 200 bpm). I don't exercise much in this zone, because as a competitive athlete I need to spend most of my workout time at higher intensities to get the high-performance results I'm looking for. This doesn't mean the Healthy Heart zone isn't important. For most people it's absolutely vital, and their first step on the road to their new lives.

My friend Amy had tried the standard yo-yo exercise programs for the last ten years. Each January she got motivated to start an exercise program, and by February she had always fallen off the wagon. This past January, after getting a heart rate monitor for a holiday gift, she took the first steps to her new life: fifteen minutes on an indoor exercise bike three times per week in her Healthy Heart zone. For the first time in her life, March and April arrived and she was still exercising. Finally she had found an exercise program that was fun and easy, and provided the benefits she wanted: a stronger heart, stable weight, more energy (because her blood pressure was dropping), and better muscle tone.

On the other end of the spectrum, some people exercise regularly but don't know how to exercise the right amount. Take my brother Chris. An avid runner for the last five years, he recently found out he has high blood pressure. Fortunately, his family doctor knew about Heart Zone Training and prescribed a change in Chris's exercise program. After convincing Chris to start measuring his heart rate, the doctor instructed him to do all of his exercising in the 50 to 60 percent Healthy Heart zone. In eight weeks Chris's blood pressure dropped twenty points, and he was able to go off his medication. It turned out that Chris had been exercising too hard for too long and had actually been hurting his health.

There are four zones beyond the Healthy Heart zone, each of which provides different benefits. The next zone up from the Healthy Heart zone in intensity is the Temperate zone at 60 to 70 percent of your Max HR. Here you will burn the highest percentage of your calories as fat. If you're out of shape, and getting in shape is your goal, then you should spend most of your exercise time in this zone. Since my body contains little body fat in relation to my muscles, I don't work out in this zone. But my friend Sandy, who has been on a merry-go-round of diets over the years, has shed (and kept off!) eighteen unwanted pounds by cycling thirty minutes every other day at 60 to 70 percent of her Max HR of 150. By monitoring her heart rate every few minutes, she can maintain an average heart rate of 90 to 105 bpm and burn off a lot of fat calories.

Above the Temperate zone is the Aerobic zone, where you maintain 70 to 80 percent of your Max HR. Most people feel exhilarated exercising in the Aerobic zone, because here they realize the benefits of improved breathing and blood circulation, breaking a sweat, working harder, and feeling generally more fit. For people exercising to maintain all-around fitness, this zone makes the most sense. Walter Bingham, retired from sports writing at age sixty-two, loves to play tennis and golf; he also runs some fifteen miles a week. He finds the Aerobic zone perfect for his needs, getting his heart rate between 119 and 136 bpm (70 to 80 percent of his Max HR of 170) for twenty minutes, three times weekly.

The next zone, the Anaerobic or Threshold zone, takes you through a doorway into a new world of training, where you cross over the border from aerobic to anaerobic exercise. During anaerobic workouts, the body's muscles, including the heart, have gone beyond the aerobic state, where they consume lots of oxygen, to a threshold beyond which the body cannot supply enough oxygen. This is where athletes say they "feel the burn." I work out in this zone a lot, for short periods of time, exercising at 80 to 90 percent of my Max HR of 200 (from 160 to 180 bpm). You can only stay in this zone for a limited amount of time because your body will protect itself from over-work and slow you down if you keep it up too long. Within this zone, however, the competitive athlete gains tremendous performance benefits.

The final zone, the Redline zone, is an anaerobic state that taxes your breathing and muscles to their utmost. Kurt, a world-class marathoner, can stay in this zone for only a few minutes at 90 percent of his 195 bpm Max HR (176 bpm) and only for a few seconds at 100 percent of his Max HR. This is not a zone you will probably select, unless, like Kurt, you are already a superb physical specimen engaged in the highest levels of professional competition. It's called Redline because of the obvious dangers it presents for the average person. It's a hot time in the Redline zone.

Choosing Zones

What about those of us—the majority, probably—who would like to get a variety of results from the time we spend on our bikes, stair-steppers, or local trails? We don't have to just pick one zone and stay with it forever, do we?

Of course not. People change their fitness programs all the time, adjusting them to their current needs and desires. In fact, it's better to start out with a varied program. You'll be gaining a variety of benefits while keeping yourself from getting bored with the same old routine.

Suppose you're the typical thirty-year-old who is neither totally out of shape nor really in shape, not really over-weight, but not as slim as you'd like to be. You could benefit most from Heart Zone Training by mixing up your exercise routine, working out in a variety of zones, perhaps the Healthy Heart zone on Monday, the Temperate zone on Wednesday, and the Aerobic zone on Friday. A less stren-uous activity such as walking could fill your Monday workout needs, while a stationary bike and an aerobics class might better suit your Wednesday and Friday workouts. Next week, vary the pattern, if you can. Even if you never bother with the Threshold or Redline zones, you'll still be strength-ening your heart, improving your figure, and enhancing your aerobic endurance. No more puffing up the stairs for you!

What about the forty-year-old fitness buff, running him-self ragged trying to keep his competitive edge for the next Ironman Triathlon? The Healthy Heart and Temperate zones wouldn't do much for him, it's true. But at the same time, he's probably spending too much time in the Threshold zone and not enough in the Aerobic zone. Rebalancing his workout intensities might actually make his occasional forays into the Redline zone more effective. He won't feel so burned out by overworking his body with too much time in the Threshold zone.

How about the fifty-year-old man who's been caught by middle-age spread, whose teenage addiction to french fries has really caught up with him, who hasn't exercised since he played golf on a trip to Florida two years ago? He would do well to emphasize the Healthy Heart zone but to do, say, every third workout in the Temperate zone—at least until he and his doctor are sure he is ready to try something as stren-uous as the Aerobic zone.

What about someone older, sixty-five or so, who has never had much of a problem with her weight but who is beginning to feel she needs a little more vim and vigor? The Healthy Heart zone may be all she needs, and there's nothing wrong with that, either.

The point is, Heart Zone Training is what you make of it. Once you figure out your needs, then choosing your training intensity—your zone(s)—comes naturally. In the next chapter you'll customize your own initial thirty-day program. But for the time being, keep in mind that once you've committed yourself to a fitness-based lifestyle, you can adapt the principles of Heart Zone Training to your specific needs now and for the rest of your life.

FITness

Having gotten into the habit of measuring your heart rate, either manually (pulse rate) or mechanically (a heart rate monitor), and, having figured out your personal fitness goals and the corresponding heart rate zones, you're ready to work out. Now the big question is "How much?" To answer that question, you should consider your personal "FIT":

F stands for frequency—how many times per week you should exercise.

I stands for intensity—in what heart rate zone(s) you should exercise.

T stands for time—how long or how many minutes you should exercise each workout session.

When doctors give a prescription for medicine, they do so precisely. There's no confusion about what, how, and when. Unfortunately, we can't do that with exercise programs. (If we tried, we'd be losing all the benefits of customizing goals and results.) Most people don't realize that no two people, even of the same age, sex, and fitness, respond the same way to exercise. Determining your exercise prescription (your FIT) depends on a lot of other factors: where you live, the work you do, health problems such as a bad back, and everything else that makes you a unique individual.

However, a few rules of thumb generally apply:

- Don't overdo it. You've heard the expression, "No pain, no gain." That's hogwash. If you suddenly go from running a comfortable few miles to entering a marathon, you'll most likely hurt yourself. If you haven't exercised routinely for a year or more, almost any strenuous workout will cause some pain, and nothing undermines your commitment more than sore, aching muscles.

- Do *do* it. I've never met anyone who hasn't done some sort of exercise in his or her life. Start there. If walking or jogging or bicycling or climbing stairs bores you, try something new: weight training, tennis, swimming, yoga, karate, tap dancing. In addition to getting fit, you might also pick up a whole new hobby!

- Take your time. Although you will see concrete results by the end of the first week of your initial thirty-day program, you'll see even more at the end of the month. Remember, you're committed to a long-range, not a short-range, goal: a lifetime of fitness.

- Take your heart rate. I don't want to sound like a saleswoman, but I've found that the new, inexpensive heart rate monitors add an interesting dimension to any workout. A good tennis racquet costs over a hundred dollars, and home exercise equipment such as rowing machines and stationary bikes can cost several hundred. An investment in a heart rate monitor can pay handsome returns, keeping you continuously, effortlessly, and accurately on your Heart Zone Training goals. For more about buying a monitor, turn to the appendix, "Choosing a Heart Rate Monitor."

For relatively unfit people beginning Heart Zone Training, these guidelines also apply:

- Frequency for the novice heart zone trainer: three to four times per week.
- Intensity for the novice heart zone trainer: 50 to 60 percent of Max HR (the Healthy Heart zone).
- Time for the novice heart zone trainer: fifteen to twenty minutes per workout.

If you start in the most comfortable zone for short periods of time, you'll find yourself enjoying every minute of it, and you'll be eager to push for more. That's great, but please be careful. You may end up doing more than you should too early in your program. Try to keep in mind the three P's: Passion, Patience, and Perseverance. Give your body time to adjust and the activities it loves (Passion), move up gradually (Patience), and stick to your program (Perseverance). Guess I left out the fourth P—Progression. When you do the first three, you get the fourth for free.

Before You Start

Before starting any exercise program, you should follow the prudent guidelines of the American College of Sports Medicine. Here is a brief synopsis of those recommendations:

Apparently healthy men over age forty and apparently healthy women over age fifty should have a medical examination and diagnostic exercise test before starting a vigorous exercise program, as should symptomatic men and women of any age. However, these procedures are not essential when such persons begin a moderate-intensity exercise regimen.

If you aren't sure what category you're in, here's a quick and easy test. This PAR-Q (Physical Activity Readiness Questionnaire) is designed to identify those people for whom certain physical activities might be inappropriate or who should receive medical advice about the kind of activity most suitable for them. If you answer "yes" to any of the following questions, you should not start an exercise program until you get clearance from your medical doctor.

This is another reason I always advise newcomers to Heart Zone Training to start in the Healthy Heart zone—it simply poses less of a medical risk than the higher zones. With low-intensity exercise, there is less need for medical evaluation and program supervision or monitoring.

ARE YOU READY TO START AN EXERCISE PROGRAM?

If you're thinking of starting (or intensifying) an exercise program, the best first step is to ask yourself the questions listed below, which are designed to help you determine whether increased exercise could prove hazardous. For most people, starting a new program shouldn't present a problem. These questions will help you determine whether you are one of the small number of adults for whom exercise might cause health problems and who should consult with a medical professional before starting a new program. Answer the following questions honestly:

YES	NO	
❏	❏	1. Has your doctor told you that you have heart trouble?
❏	❏	2. Do you frequently suffer from heart or chest pains?
❏	❏	3. Do you feel faint or have severe spells of dizziness?
❏	❏	4. Has your doctor ever told you that your blood pressure was too high?
❏	❏	5. Has your doctor ever told you that you have bone or joint problems such as arthritis that could be aggravated by exercise?
❏	❏	6. Are there any other physical reasons why you should not start an exercise program?
❏	❏	7. Are you over age 65 and not accustomed to vigorous exercise?

YOUR NAME: _____ TODAY'S DATE: _____

If you answered NO to all of these questions:

If you answered honestly and accurately, you are probably ready to get started on either a sound exercise program that takes your overall condition and level of fitness into account, or a fitness appraisal. (Put off starting if you have a temporary minor illness, such as a common cold.)

If you answered YES to one or more questions:

If you haven't already done so, consult your doctor before increasing your level of physical activity or taking a fitness appraisal. Tell your doctor which questions you answered YES to and give him or her a copy of this questionnaire.

After your doctor has evaluated your situation, ask him or her whether you can start a program of unrestricted physical activity that begins easily and progresses gradually, or whether you should stay with restricted or supervised activity that meets your specific needs (at least to start).

Adapted from the PAR-Q Physical Activation Readiness Questionnaire developed by the British Columbia Ministry of Health.

Your Personal Log

As you work through this book, you should be logging important numbers that relate to Heart Zone Training. You'll find a Personal Heart Zone Training Log at the end of each chapter. Take some time now, before you begin Chapter 2, to fill out the log below.

MY HEART RATE ZONES

1. Resting Heart Rate (before getting out of bed in the morning):
   _____ bpm

2. Ambient Heart Rate (while sitting comfortably and quietly):
   _____ bpm

3. Maximum Heart Rate (using one of the SubMax tests):
   _____ bpm

4. My Heart Rate Zones

Healthy Heart (50–60 percent Max HR)	_____ bpm to	_____ bpm
Temperate (60–70 percent Max HR)	_____ bpm to	_____ bpm
Aerobic (70–80 percent Max HR)	_____ bpm to	_____ bpm
Threshold (80–90 percent Max HR)	_____ bpm to	_____ bpm
Redline (90–100 percent Max HR)	_____ bpm to	_____ bpm

Designing an Initial Thirty-Day Program

Patented, by-the-book, one-size-fits-all diet, exercise, and fitness programs have always bugged me. My career as an endurance athlete and fitness educator has definitely taught me one thing: No two people share exactly the same physical characteristics, lifestyles, and exercise needs and goals. Take my friends Jennifer and Wendy, for instance.

They called me recently to ask some questions that had arisen a month after they attended one of my Heart Zone Training seminars. Jennifer works as an engineer for a Silicon Valley computer company, and Wendy is an aerobics instructor at a health club in San Jose. Though they are roommates and spend a lot of time together, their lives are very different.

Not having exercised regularly for some years, and wanting to shed some excess weight, Jennifer had wisely started her Heart Zone Training program in the Healthy Heart and Temperate zones. Since she already owned a stationary home exercise bike, she worked out on it for fifteen-minute periods three times a week, keeping track of her heart rate with a heart rate monitor. "I'm seeing some results," she told me on the phone. "At first it was a lot of effort to train for the fifteen minutes, and my heart rate would keep on getting too high for the Temperate zone, breaking through my ceiling of 70 percent Max HR. Now, training for fifteen minutes is pretty easy, and my heart rate doesn't drift out of the zone as often. Does that sound all right?"

Yes, I told her, she had begun to develop a healthier, less hard-working heart. If she wanted, she could now try increasing her time on the bike, and maybe increase her intensity, too. "But Sally," she protested, "it's so boring. I'm not sure I can stick with it. What can I do?"

Jennifer had hit the motivation wall. So many beginning exercisers start out with all the commitment in the world to achieving their goals, but then, after they start to see results, they get bored with the routine and quit. Jennifer had not, as I told her, really designed a *personal program* she could enjoy and maintain with enthusiasm.

Wendy, on the other hand, had been quite fit before she started Heart Zone Training. She began her program with the intention of working out mostly in the Aerobic zone, with the occasional session in the Threshold zone. However, during the last month she had run five miles in her Aerobic and Threshold zones three times a week, taught her aerobics class three days a week with thirty minutes of swimming afterward, and played racquetball twice a week with her boyfriend. "I don't know, Sally," she said. "I've noticed that my resting heart rate has actually *increased* by almost five beats per minute since I've been on the program, which seems strange, and I'm really tired all the time. What's wrong?"

Wendy had run herself into the overtraining wall, something that happens fairly often when serious fitness buffs start Heart Zone Training with a vengeance. She too had failed to design a *personal program* that fit the requirements of her lifestyle and her existing workout schedule. She was working too hard too long.

I recommend you take a few lessons from Jennifer and Wendy's awkward Heart Zone Training beginnings as you set about creating your own initial four-week program:

- Begin realistically and gradually, working out in one or two zones during the first weeks.
- Incorporate different activities into your training so you won't hit the motivational wall.
- Avoid the overtraining wall and don't try to do too many workouts each week, especially in the higher-intensity zones.
- Listen to your body—if you feel pain or tiredness, back off to a lower zone.
- Keep in mind that your initial program will turn into a ninety-day program, then a program for a lifetime, so don't expect too much (or too little) by the end of the first month.

Throughout my life in sports and business, I have come to believe that all success depends on those same three P's: Passion, Perseverance, and Patience. You must feel passionate about living a healthier life, and nothing will fuel that passion more than enjoyment of the process of training and making measurable improvements in fitness. This is where variety in your activities and heart rate monitoring come in.

You must also persevere, never letting setbacks such as illness or boredom stay in your way. This is where creating a personalized first-four-week program comes in. And you must be patient as you create your new life, your new *you*. One month may seem like an eternity at the beginning of your Heart Zone Training, but a few months or years from now it will look like a brief, though important, moment in your life. Now, before you embark on the next step on that lifetime journey, I want you to revisit the FIT factors that should be your guides every step of the way.

FIT Revisited

In Chapter 1 we talked about FIT: frequency, intensity, and time. As you build your initial four-week program, you will want to increase all these components of your workout gradually, week by week.

At this point, let's assume you have been experimenting with various exercises and measuring their effects on your heart rate. Let's say you have been working out with a frequency of three times per week at an intensity of 50 to 60 percent of your Max HR and for not less than fifteen minutes per workout. You know your resting, ambient, and Max HR, you have calculated your five heart rate zones, and you're getting comfortable measuring your heart rate manually or with a heart rate monitor. Now you're ready to formalize your first week of Heart Zone Training.

Over the course of the next 4 weeks you will slowly increase each of the three FIT factors, first boosting your workout frequency from three times a week to four, then adding five minutes to your time-in-zone, moving from fifteen minutes to twenty per workout while adding another fifteen-minute workout to the weekly schedule. By the end of the first month you will gradually have increased your overall time-in-zone to the point where you are regularly doing twenty-five-minute workouts. In addition you'll go from spending most of your time in one zone to spending half there and half in a higher intensity zone.

Of course, you'll be tailoring your program to your own unique physical characteristics, lifestyle, needs, and goals. As I guide you through this process, however, I'll be using Jennifer, the unfit engineer, and Wendy, the fit aerobics instructor, to illustrate key points. Let's do it!

Week 1

Jennifer's personal log from Chapter 1 looks like this:

Resting HR: 61 bpm		
Ambient HR: 72 bpm		
Max HR: 163 bpm		
Heart Rate Zones	**Floor**	**Ceiling**
Healthy Heart:	81	98 bpm
Temperate:	98	114 bpm
Aerobic:	114	130 bpm
Threshold:	130	146 bpm
Redline:	146	163 bpm

Given Jennifer's lack of regular exercise and her twenty pounds of excess weight, she will want to start her first week by increasing her frequency of workouts from three to four, spending most of her time in the Healthy Heart Zone at around 90 bpm but occasionally pushing into the Temperate zone at around 105 bpm.

To avoid the motivational wall, Jennifer should add another enjoyable activity to her exercise bike routine, perhaps taking a brisk fifteen-minute walk twice a week. Her Week 1 log might look like this:

JENNIFER WEEK 1	SUNDAY	MONDAY	TUESDAY	WEDNESDAY	THURSDAY	FRIDAY	SATURDAY	WEEKLY SUMMARY
ACTIVITY	Walk	Rest	Bike	Rest	Walk	Rest	Bike	2 activities
FREQUENCY	1		1		1		1	4 workouts
INTENSITY	Healthy Heart		Temperate		Healthy Heart		Temperate	2 zones
TIME	15 minutes		15 minutes		15 minutes		15 minutes	60 minutes

At this point Jennifer may be wondering how she will find the time to continue to work out so frequently. Exercise researchers have asked a lot of busy people this question and have found an answer: Those people who set a specific time to exercise each day enjoy a higher success rate than those who decide each day at random what time to work out. They call this phenomenon "exercise compliance." The researchers also discovered that people tend to exercise more consistently if they train in the morning. It seems that busy people will sacrifice exercise time later in the day when they're tired and caught up in other obligations.

"Great," moans Jennifer, "now I can get bored *four* times a week, instead of three" My advice to Jennifer is to invite Wendy or some other friend to join in her walks. Researchers have also learned that people who train with a friend exercise more regularly than the solo trainer. It really helps to exercise with a buddy as often as possible. For one thing, if you make arrangements with someone else, you'll be less likely to change your mind about going out to exercise. You'll also enjoy yourself more. Your weekend workouts, for example, might include your partner or other family member—it's a good way to spend time together. During the week, when you may have to fit your workouts into a hectic work schedule, invite a business colleague to join you or make a point of going to a local fitness club or recreation center before work. One sixty-one-year-old I know likes to walk from her office to a local coffee shop three-quarters of a mile away each weekday morning for her cup of decaf. That way she's consistently motivated to get going and stay going for about half an hour a day, five days a week.

We need to pause here for a moment and talk a little more about time. Bear in mind that when we talk about time, we're actually talking about three different things.

1. *What is the total length of the workout?* Here I'm talking about all the actual time spent moving your body. This includes time spent warming up and cooling down. For example, perhaps you started out with fifteen-minute Healthy Heart zone workouts. In reality a fifteen-minute low-intensity workout is going to take you closer to twenty minutes, accounting for the time you spend getting into, then getting out of, the zone as you warm up and cool down by exercising gently. Since we are moving toward twenty-five-minute workouts, we have to figure, for the Healthy Heart zone at least, that they will actually take about thirty minutes of our time.

2. *How much time during each workout do I spend in my exercise zone?* When I think about how time relates to my workouts, I'm usually concerned with my "time-in-zone," or TIZ. **This is what really matters in Heart Zone Training: how much time you actually spend in the zone, not including warming up or cooling down.** For a

Healthy Heart workout, for example, since getting into your personal zone doesn't require much increase in effort, you may only spend a minute or two exercising before you get into the zone and another couple of minutes cooling down out of the zone. For a Redline session, however, you may spend ten minutes getting ready for your one minute in the zone, then another ten minutes cooling down again.

Why am I interested in these different numbers? Because the amount of time you spend in each of the zones determines in large part how much benefit you are going to receive from that time.

Keep in mind that you don't have to make all your workouts the same length. It obviously makes sense for more intense workouts to be briefer than lower-intensity ones, for example. It also might make sense for you to have a single longer workout session on the weekend, then three shorter ones during the week. Frank, a forty-five-year-old lawyer, can sometimes manage to pull enough time out of his weekdays to do extended sessions, but mostly he has to settle for a twenty-minute swim before work here, a thirty-minute walk there. On the weekends, though, he really looks forward to spending an hour playing tennis on one or both days.

3. *How much of my overall week's workout time do I spend in any given zone?* In other words, now that I'm about to start doing multiple-zone weeks, how do I want to divide up my time? Is the Healthy Heart zone more important to my goals, or the Temperate zone? Do I want to break up my time fifty-fifty or give only a quarter of my time to the higher-intensity zone? In the weekly plans that follow I've made these decisions for you, but after you complete your first month of training, you'll be answering such questions for yourself and shaping your workout plans accordingly.

Let's return to Wendy, the fit aerobics instructor whose personal log looks like this:

Resting HR: 50 bpm

Ambient HR: 63 bpm

Max HR: 185 bpm

Heart Rate Zones	Floor	Ceiling
Healthy Heart:	93	111 bpm
Temperate:	111	130 bpm
Aerobic:	130	148 bpm
Threshold:	148	166 bpm
Redline:	166	185 bpm

Because she has worked out regularly for many years, and because she feels tempted to overdo her Heart Zone Training and drive herself into the overtraining wall, Wendy should launch her first week of the program *without* increasing the frequency, intensity, or time of her workouts. Instead, her first week's main goal should be to learn to monitor her heart rate much more closely than in the past and to keep herself within set heart rate zones for each of her workouts, instead of passing in and out of them at random as she pushes herself or becomes tired during a training bout. Wendy will focus on working out primarily in the Aerobic zone at around 140 bpm, with occasional, controlled forays up into the Threshold zone around 155 bpm. The key for Wendy is not to overdo it. Regular, moderate training, with limited higher-intensity exercise, should be her strategy. And Wendy might also learn to take a day off from training each week, to give her body a chance to rejuvenate itself for the next week's activities. Her Week 1 log might look like this:

WENDY WEEK 1	SUNDAY	MONDAY	TUESDAY	WEDNESDAY	THURSDAY	FRIDAY	SATURDAY	WEEKLY SUMMARY
ACTIVITY	Rest	Aerobics	Run	Racquetball	Aerobics	Swim	Aerobics	4 activities
FREQUENCY		1	1	1	1	1	1	6 workouts
INTENSITY		Aerobic	Aerobic	Temperate	Aerobic	Threshold	Aerobic	3 zones
TIME		30 minutes	30 minutes	60 minutes	30 minutes	20 minutes	30 minutes	200 minutes

"Wait a minute," Wendy might object, "I thought the whole idea was for me to get into better shape. I'm actually cutting down on my workouts." Yes and no. Yes, this first week will trim Wendy's exercise program a bit, so she won't feel so beat by Sunday morning. No, she's not taking a step backward fitness-wise, just because she's no longer pushing herself to (or past) her limits. Over time, Wendy will find this more sensible program evolving as she listens more closely to her body (her heart rate) and uses what she learns to help her body (and her heart) grow stronger. In less time she will actually derive greater benefits.

Your own physical condition, lifestyle, needs, and goals may parallel Wendy's or Jennifer's, or you may fall somewhere in between. If you are unfit when you begin Heart Zone Training, you should spend 100 percent of your time in the Healthy Heart zone, where you will gain two tangible benefits. Without pushing yourself to dangerous levels, you will be exercising enough to make a difference in your conditioning and to allow you to move upward over time; and you will experience a physiological result in improved cardiovascular fitness. You'll have a healthier heart.

With enhanced cardiovascular fitness, your heart can deliver more blood more efficiently and with fewer beats per minute. Your heart is strengthened, and your arteries and veins, over the long term, kept clear of fatty deposits. From the Healthy Heart zone you can also decrease your blood pressure, improve your cholesterol ratios, and stabilize or lose some body fat. If you are keeping careful track of your heart rates, you will also find that working out in the Healthy Heart zone results in lower resting and ambient heart rates. That's good.

Later on you can add an additional zone to your training to increase your workout variety and to get some additional fitness results. In the Temperate zone you'll increase your pace or workload to 60 to 70 percent of your Max HR. You will also burn a high percentage of fat calories as a source of your energy. In the Temperate zone you begin to push yourself a little harder, maybe breaking a sweat. Depending on their degree of unfitness, most folks will find Temperate zone workouts somewhat easy to somewhat challenging.

I know of many people who focus all their workout time in these two zones. Combining a weight management program in the Temperate zone with heart-strengthening exercise is right on target for the needs of most busy adults. There's very little risk of injury at these intensities, for one thing, and risk is something the parent or business person can little afford. Sarah is a thirty-one-year-old freelance writer with no time to develop any interest in competitive sports or even in getting herself "all sweaty in the middle of the day," as she puts it. She's found that the Healthy Heart and Temperate zones can fit in with her lifestyle—a walk here, a bike ride there, a little light use of her rowing machine at home—while keeping the pounds off and her concerns about cardiovascular fitness in check.

If you see yourself as too fit to be working out in the lower zones, fine. Just take a cue from Wendy and be patient. You'll eventually be rewarded by progress, provided you retain your passion for fitness and persevere into Week 2 of your initial program.

Week 2

If, after Week 1, you say, "Wow, this isn't as easy as I thought—it's hard to stay within my zones and to find time to train," then you should probably continue with the Week 1 program during your second week, and not try to make any changes. If, however, you feel comfortable with your Week 1 FIT and are ready for more, you will now want to increase your time-in-zone, and maybe your workout frequency, even if you want to leave the intensity the same.

Jennifer, the out-of-shape engineer, has been gaining cardiovascular or Healthy Heart zone benefits, as well as the fat-burning benefits of the Temperate zone, during Week 1. For Week 2 she decides to increase her total workout time and add a little more variety to her workout activities. Her Week 2 log looks like this:

JENNIFER WEEK 2	SUNDAY	MONDAY	TUESDAY	WEDNESDAY	THURSDAY	FRIDAY	SATURDAY	WEEKLY SUMMARY
ACTIVITY	Tennis	Rest	Bike	Rest	Walk	Rest	Bike	3 activities
FREQUENCY	1		1		1		1	4 workouts
INTENSITY	Healthy Heart		Temperate		Healthy Heart		Temperate	2 zones
TIME	40 minutes		20 minutes		20 minutes		20 minutes	100 minutes

In Week 1 Jennifer exercised a total of sixty minutes. In Week 2 she will exercise for a total of 100 minutes. This may sound like a big jump, but she actually increased her time fairly by gradually adding only five minutes a workout to her cycling and walking routines. The big increase is the forty-minute doubles tennis session, something she'd been meaning to take up again. It's not a very strenuous activity, but Jennifer is adding variety to her program, and that should help her avoid crashing into the motivational wall. She's focusing on her goals and staying in the right zones to achieve them, getting the maximum out of each minute of exercise. After all, 100 minutes is less time than it takes to watch a video on Friday night; in fact, depending on the traffic, it can be less time than it takes to drive to the store, choose a video, stand in line, and drive back again!

If you were in poorer shape than Jennifer before you started the Heart Zone Training program, you should be prepared for the experience of working out at a higher intensity. Even though you're starting with only fifteen minutes in the Temperate zone, those fifteen minutes can be a little demanding. In the Temperate zone you'll likely sweat a little, but you shouldn't get short of breath. If you do find yourself starting to feel overwhelmed by the intensity, stop and manually take your pulse or check the numbers on your heart rate monitor. You could very likely have gone out of the Temperate zone and into the Aerobic zone; easily done, but we're not ready for that yet.

Wendy, on the other hand, feels more than ready to increase the intensity of her workouts, so she adds double-zone workouts. She designs Week 2 like this:

WENDY WEEK 2	SUNDAY	MONDAY	TUESDAY	WEDNESDAY	THURSDAY	FRIDAY	SATURDAY	WEEKLY SUMMARY
ACTIVITY	Rest	Aerobics	Run	Racquetball	Aerobics	Swim	Aerobics	4 activities
FREQUENCY		1	1	1	1	1	1	6 workouts
INTENSITY		Aerobic (25 minutes) Threshold (5 minutes)	Aerobic (30 minutes) Threshold (10 minutes)	Temperate	Aerobic (25 minutes) Threshold (5 minutes)	Aerobic (10 minutes) Threshold (20 minutes)	Aerobic (25 minutes) Threshold (5 minutes)	3 zones
TIME		30 minutes	40 minutes	60 minutes	30 minutes	30 minutes	30 minutes	220 minutes

She's added ten minutes to each of her running and swimming workouts, but more importantly, she's added time at a higher intensity, in the Threshold zone, to each of her Aerobic zone workouts. Wendy has done this by splitting the time of each of these workouts among two zones, a double-zoner. She spends the majority of her time in the Aerobic zone but adds a few minutes in the Threshold zone after she's well warmed up. These few minutes may not seem like a lot, but she will probably feel the difference in her muscles soon afterward and in her overall fitness in the future. If Wendy finds herself hitting the overtraining wall, she should back off a bit.

As you design your own Week 2, do so in a way that suits your present physical condition, your needs, and your goals. Jennifer and Wendy are ambitious and can find the increased time to train. Your own program should parallel theirs only on principle: You too want to do more each week, but you want to do it in a way that fits in with your lifestyle and doesn't cause you boredom or pain.

Week 3

Whatever your starting point, if you stick with your program for a couple of weeks, you are going to be champing at the bit for more time in higher zones, as your workouts feel increasingly easier. Your body is adapting to the increases in workload (higher-intensity zones for longer durations) by getting fitter, and to keep on feeling that you're putting out the same amount of effort, you're going to need to increase the intensity and/or duration of each workout. So during Week 3 you may want to add either another, higher-intensity, zone or more time to the existing zones in your schedule. How will you do it? Gradually and patiently, of course.

Let's look at Jennifer's Week 3 log:

JENNIFER WEEK 3	SUNDAY	MONDAY	TUESDAY	WEDNESDAY	THURSDAY	FRIDAY	SATURDAY	WEEKLY SUMMARY
ACTIVITY	Walk	Rest	Bike	Tennis	Walk	Rest	Bike	3 activities
FREQUENCY	1		1	1	1		1	5 workouts
INTENSITY	Healthy Heart (15 minutes) Temperate (10 minutes)		Temperate	Healthy Heart (20 minutes) Temperate (20 minutes)	Healthy Heart (15 minutes) Temperate (10 minutes)		Temperate	2 zones
TIME	25 minutes		25 minutes	40 minutes	25 minutes		25 minutes	140 minutes

The first thing you may notice is that Jennifer has increased her training frequency from four times a week to five. She's been feeling good, has dropped a couple of pounds, and has been eager to move ahead. Her body's been giving her unmistakable messages that it's gotten comfortable and is ready to move on. This increase in frequency, combined with an increase in her minimum workout time by five minutes (from twenty minutes to twenty-five), means that she is now working out for 140 minutes a week. Another change Jennifer made was to pick up the pace of her walks and add some Temperate zone time to each of them. She also tried switching her doubles tennis game for a singles match, knowing that would increase the intensity of her workout.

Wendy probably shouldn't increase the frequency of her workouts—getting burned out or injured is too real a possibility for someone who trains as much as she does—but she is eager to increase the time of her runs and swims and the intensity of her racquetball session, now that she's comfortable with the game. Here's her Week 3 log:

WENDY WEEK 3	SUNDAY	MONDAY	TUESDAY	WEDNESDAY	THURSDAY	FRIDAY	SATURDAY	WEEKLY SUMMARY
ACTIVITY	Rest	Aerobics	Run	Racquetball	Aerobics	Swim	Aerobics	4 activities
FREQUENCY		1	1	1	1	1	1	6 workouts
INTENSITY		Aerobic (25 minutes) Threshold (5 minutes)	Aerobic (40 minutes) Threshold (18 minutes) Redline (2 minutes)	Temperate (45 minutes) Aerobic (15 minutes)	Aerobic (25 minutes) Threshold (5 minutes)	Aerobic (20 minutes) Threshold (18 minutes) Redline (2 minutes)	Aerobic (25 minutes) Threshold (5 minutes)	4 zones
TIME		30 minutes	60 minutes	60 minutes	30 minutes	40 minutes	30 minutes	250 minutes

Wendy's adding a total of thirty minutes to her week's training time, as well as making small adjustments to her training intensities, shifting up the difficulty where she can. The urge to push herself harder is still strong, however, and

Wendy gives in to the impulse during her run and swim and goes all-out for a few minutes into the Redline zone. Her heart rate monitor allows her to pinpoint feedback she needs to make sure she's in the Redline for only two minutes each time. Unless you are in peak condition coming into Heart Zone Training, there is no way you should try to push yourself into the Redline zone during your initial four-week program. Even the Threshold and Aerobic zones may be beyond your reach for the time being.

Week 4

I call this week the Heart Zone plateau, because after you've spent three weeks increasing the frequency, intensity, and time of your workouts, it's usually a good idea to settle in and pull the maximum benefits from the third week's agenda. Don't worry, in the chapters ahead we'll be looking at plenty of additional ways to manage your weight, strengthen your heart, and increase your fitness and speed. We'll also be designing a ninety-day program to incorporate all aspects of your own Heart Zone Training.

Jennifer and Wendy may use their Week 3 logs for Week 4, though both will make minor adjustments based on their experiences over the past weeks. Jennifer, for example, finds singles tennis a bit too tiring during the middle of the week and moves that activity to Saturday. You've got to make adjustments to make it all fit together. Then she decides to replace one exercise bike workout by joining a beginner's aerobics class, because the bike still bores her and Wendy has been trying to talk her into aerobics for months now. Her Week 4 log looks like this:

Sally Edwards' Heart Zone Training

JENNIFER WEEK 4	SUNDAY	MONDAY	TUESDAY	WEDNESDAY	THURSDAY	FRIDAY	SATURDAY	WEEKLY SUMMARY
ACTIVITY	Walk	Rest	Bike	Aerobics	Walk	Rest	Tennis	4 activities
FREQUENCY	1		1	1	1		1	5 workouts
INTENSITY	Healthy Heart (15 minutes) Temperate (10 minutes)		Temperate	Healthy Heart (10 minutes) Temperate (10 minutes) Aerobic (10 minutes)	Healthy Heart (15 minutes) Temperate (10 minutes)		Healthy Heart (20 minutes) Temperate (20 minutes)	3 zones
TIME	25 minutes		25 minutes	30 minutes	25 minutes		40 minutes	145 minutes

Unable to set aside another day for working out, Jennifer has decided to stick with five workouts per week. However, she has been feeling so energized, she has set her sights on moving into the Aerobic zone, which she does during her Wednesday class for a brief, manageable, ten minutes a session. Otherwise, Jennifer's Week 4 log is simply a fine-tuning of her Week 3 schedule.

Wendy does pretty much the same, but having found that those four minutes in the Redline zone have slammed her into the overtraining wall, she backs off into the Threshold zone, causing her to adjust her Week 4 log slightly:

WENDY WEEK 4	SUNDAY	MONDAY	TUESDAY	WEDNESDAY	THURSDAY	FRIDAY	SATURDAY	WEEKLY SUMMARY
ACTIVITY	Rest	Aerobics	Run	Racquetball	Aerobics	Swim	Aerobics	4 activities
FREQUENCY		1	1	1	1	1	1	6 workouts
INTENSITY		Aerobic (25 minutes) Threshold (5 minutes)	Aerobic (40 minutes) Threshold (20 minutes)	Temperate (45 minutes) Aerobic (15 minutes)	Aerobic (25 minutes) Threshold (5 minutes)	Aerobic (20 minutes) Threshold (20 minutes)	Aerobic (25 minutes) Threshold (5 minutes)	3 zones
TIME		30 minutes	60 minutes	60 minutes	30 minutes	40 minutes	30 minutes	250 minutes

You know those transparent human-body models that biology teachers use to show what goes on inside people? Imagine that we could look inside Jennifer's and Wendy's bodies and minds after Week 4 of their initial Heart Zone Training program. What would we see?

- A stronger heart muscle that works more efficiently and contracts more fully and a cardiovascular system with fewer fatty deposits
- Better skeletal muscle tone that enables the body to do more work with less effort
- An enhanced muscle-to-body-fat ratio and an overall loss of excess fat
- A healthy and normal appetite that fuels the body efficiently without adding unwanted pounds
- A rosier complexion and an all-around healthier appearance
- A broad smile that broadcasts a sense of accomplishment and satisfaction over having embarked on a lifetime of fitness
- A happier outlook on life, greater self-esteem, an energized, confident state of well-being

These same benefits come to all heart zone trainers, from those who begin their programs at ground zero to those who participate regularly in athletic competition. Before we leave our four-week program, let's take a look now at both ends of the spectrum.

If, in Chapter 1, you classified yourself as being in poor-to-average shape, you'll want to figure out what kinds of activities fit into the lower zones you'll be working out in. For example, should you be walking or running, cycling or swimming, doing aerobic dance or square dance, circuit training or weight lifting, golf or basketball? Heart Zone Training is universal, so it really doesn't matter what specific activity you do. What matters is that you keep your heart rate at a level appropriate for the zone you wish to work out in for the benefit you want to achieve.

It's far too easy to train above or below your selected zone, and the only foolproof way to catch yourself is by measuring your heart rate. So if you want to know "Should I jog or should I walk?" the answer is that it depends on you. To stay within the Temperate zone some may need to walk quite slowly because of their current lack of cardiovascular conditioning. Those who are fitter may have to jog to exert enough effort to keep their heart's workload or intensity within the desired range.

Following are a few workout suggestions for the zones the person in poor-to-average shape will be training in during the first four weeks. You are in no way limited to these, however. If you find that your heart rate is sufficiently elevated by vacuuming, for example, to qualify that activity as a Temperate zone workout, by all means, go for it! (Note: If you are looking for more details on any of the following activities, check ahead to Chapter 3, "Getting and Keeping a Healthy Heart," and Chapter 4, "Managing Your Weight," where we describe these workouts in more detail.) The following suggestions apply to the Jennifers of the world:

Suggested Healthy Heart Zone Activities

- Walking: Whether you walk steadily or briskly will depend on your heart rate numbers. The more unconditioned may need to go for a steady walk, not a brisk stride. And don't forget that for variety, walking outdoors one day and indoors on a treadmill another will help avoid the motivational wall.

- Bicycling: It may take going very slowly, but almost everyone can do a Healthy Heart zone workout on a bike or stationary exercise bike. Don't try to ride the hills of San Francisco, though—cycling can be one of your most intense workouts.

- Swimming: You've seen the classes of sixty-, seventy-, and eighty-year-olds slowly swimming the breast stroke at your local pool. What do they know that you don't? For one thing, they know that a slow swim is a perfect Healthy Heart activity and is among the gentlest whole-body workouts possible.

- Fitness Classes: Try the floor exercise portion of a fitness class or of an aerobics class. Take care, though, to do only the floor exercise portion and not to get carried away into an actual aerobics session—that'll get your heart rate way up in a hurry. Yoga classes are essentially all floor exercise and are sometimes appropriate for the Healthy Heart zone.

- Weight Machines: A steady twenty- to thirty-minute bout of circuit training and low-resistance weight lifting is usually good for a Healthy Heart zone workout, and will certainly shape those deltoids, but check your heart rate while you're training to be sure.

Suggested Temperate Zone Activities

- Walking: Most folks can get within the Temperate zone by going for a walk, a brisk one. Race-walking will certainly do it for you, although the very best race-walkers push into and sometimes beyond their Aerobic zone on occasion. For the very fit who aren't familiar with race-walking techniques, an easy jog might be required to get their heart rates sufficiently elevated.

- Bicycling: At moderate intensities, taking a bike ride or an extended stationary bike session will get you into the Temperate zone. Take care, though, to monitor your heart rate frequently. As you tire it'll drift upward, so you may want to take it a little easier toward the end of your ride.

- Stair-Stepping: A mainstay of health clubs, although we are now seeing some more compact models for home use. Low-intensity stair-stepping can be a fun way to get into the Temperate zone. Again, though, don't try to push yourself too hard. Once your heart rate elevates out of the selected zone, you stop getting that zone's benefits.

- Swimming: Steady, freestyle swimming is either a Temperate or Aerobic zone activity, depending on how fast you try to go, how much effort you are putting out, and how good your stroke is. Gentle, steady laps are all you need to maximize your body's fat-burning abilities.

- Fitness Classes: Low-impact fitness or "aerobics" classes fit the Temperate zone bill for most moderately fit people. Continue to avoid high-impact classes at this point, since they may elevate your heart rate out of the Temperate zone. (After all, they're not called "aerobics" classes for nothing.)

- Tennis: This can be a good Temperate zone activity, but it does have one drawback, namely that for most of us the exercise isn't continuous but an interval–type workout. We stand around waiting for a ball to come our way, lob it back, then occasionally chase the ones that get past us. My suggestion is to measure your heart rate frequently during a tennis game, not only right after you've chased a ball down the street, and find out whether your heart rate stays steadily in the zone. If it does, then tennis is for you. If it doesn't, play tennis for fun and for its interval benefit—multiple zones.

What if you're in excellent shape? Happily, many of my readers will already be fit. Marlene is a thirty-five-year-old recreational marathoner with whom I train occasionally. When she and I first discussed her starting Heart Zone Training, she said she liked the idea but didn't want to stop doing her normal training sessions while she came up to speed with the new program. As a professional triathlete, I understood completely. When I was first developing Heart Zone Training, I didn't drop my daily one- to three-hour cycling, swimming, or running training sessions. What I did was experiment with the lower zones in addition to and, occasionally, instead of, my higher-intensity workouts.

Marlene went from five days a week of ten-mile runs in her Aerobic zone, to three days, then added two days of Temperate zone jogs, and one day of Threshold zone sprints or intervals. She found that with her new mix-and-match schedule of high and low zones, her energy levels stayed more even throughout the week. At the end of her first month she had lowered her marathon time by a few minutes. Marlene spent less time training and still got faster.

If you are a high-intensity competitive athlete or have an existing program, I suggest you continue with your normal training, complementing it with heart rate monitoring if you're not already doing so. However, if you want to familiarize yourself with Heart Zone Training, you should really add a few lower-intensity workouts, or switch, as Wendy did, to a deliberate thirty-day program. I think you'll be surprised to discover how it feels to train lightly again, and I think your body will thank you for it. You probably know that over-training is the most common source of injuries for those who work out.

Using heart rate monitoring for all your workouts ought to become second nature, especially if you are practicing at a competitive level for your sport. For more on using Heart Zone Training, check out Chapter 7, "Reaching the Most Advanced Level of Heart Zone Training," which I wrote specifically for athletes. In addition, both the fit and the athletic should take time to look through Chapters 5 and 6, where I discuss longer-term program development and ways to spice up your training while enhancing your fitness.

Your Personal Log

For now, weekly logs can provide a convenient way to design and adjust the frequency, intensity, and time of your initial four-week Heart Zone Training program. Fill these out week by week rather than all at once. You'll be learning a lot as you listen to your body and monitor your heart rate, and that knowledge should influence your plans for the next week.

Designing an Initial Thirty-Day Program

HEART ZONE TRAINING LOG

	SUNDAY	MONDAY	TUESDAY	WEDNESDAY	THURSDAY	FRIDAY	SATURDAY	WEEKLY SUMMARY
ACTIVITY								
FREQUENCY								
INTENSITY								
TIME								

Getting and Keeping a Healthy Heart

Recently I went with Margaret, a colleague of mine who has been recovering from a minor heart attack, for her first Heart Zone Training workout. I had determined that we would slowly walk ten minutes in one direction from our office, cross the street, and walk back the other way for ten minutes. Since Margaret needed to start out cautiously, in her Healthy Heart zone, we were supposed to take it easy, with no sweating, and we would talk the whole time we were walking to make sure she wasn't getting short of breath. Her doctor had established that Margaret's Max HR was about 170 bpm, so her Healthy Heart zone would be from 85 to 102 bpm, and that was our intensity goal.

For the first couple minutes, though, as we were warming up, we simply matched our paces. Then we glanced at the wrist displays of our heart rate monitors and compared our numbers. We saw a dramatic difference. My heart rate was 92 bpm, a little under the floor of my Healthy Heart zone of 100 to 120 bpm, meaning I would have to push myself a bit more to get into that zone. Margaret's heart rate, on the other hand, was 118 bpm, indicating that she was not only out of her Healthy Heart zone, she was actually at the top of her Temperate zone (from 102 to 119 bpm for Margaret).

That twenty-six-beat difference between her heart rate and mine illustrated the difference between a really fit heart and a really unfit one. I exercise a couple of hours a day every day, which is pretty standard for a competitive endurance athlete. Margaret was just starting to try to work out as part of her rehabilitation, and had not exercised at all in quite some time. Together we showed just how big a difference in exercise intensity there can be between two people doing the same exercise. We would never have known what effects our walk was having on us if we hadn't been measuring our heart rates. Margaret would probably have become quickly over-tired and possibly endangered her well-being, while I would have felt as if I wasn't accomplishing anything, because I wasn't exercising at a sufficient intensity to get any fitness benefits out of my time.

I immediately slowed Margaret down to below 102 bpm, the ceiling or top number for her Healthy Heart zone. When we got back to the office she said it bothered her to find her heart rate had soared so much higher than mine, but at the same time she admitted it was okay, because it showed her current fitness level in a real and measurable and accountable way. It motivated her, and because it was something she could measure, it became something she could manage.

Even with this brief exposure to Heart Zone Training, Margaret had begun the process of learning about the relationship between exercise intensity and her body's efforts. She learned what two different zones felt like and how her pace corresponded to each. She also learned that another person's pace has nothing to do with *her* exercise intensity. Margaret also found that she could breathe comfortably and didn't need to push herself through sweat and pain to achieve results that would be useful to her.

Margaret isn't the only Healthy Heart zone trainer I know, not by a long shot. Roger, a seventy-six-year-old friend of my aunt's, has just started Heart Zone Training. Now, Roger has not exactly been inactive since he retired. He fishes, plays the occasional game of golf, goes panning for gold in the Sierra foothills, and is writing a book on the history of the Sacramento region. Moreover, Roger's doctor says he's quite healthy, without the slightest symptom of any significant ailment. What inspired Roger to take the extra step of starting a regular exercise routine was the slight lessening of energy he's been feeling over the past few years. Active all his life, he wasn't about to enter his golden years lacking the vigor to do the things he enjoyed. He called his physician, who recommended regular, gentle exercise and periodic office visits to check up on his progress. It was my aunt who recommended a heart rate monitor and who arranged to introduce him to me over coffee. I gave Roger some encouragement and a few suggestions and guidelines, and he was off!

Is Your Heart a Healthy Heart?

What is a healthy heart? Part of the definition of a healthy heart is one that is able to pump out an increased volume of blood to meet increased demand. There are many ways it does this. A healthy heart, for example, squeezes more vigorously than a nonhealthy heart. A healthy heart also expands when the blood comes into the chamber, so it can take in more blood per stroke. A healthy heart contracts strongly, its valves function smoothly, and its arteries are clean and clear of fatty deposits. It also has a low resting and ambient heart rate. This means that a healthy heart can do more work and take less energy to do it.

How does a heart become healthy?

Two words: exercise and a low-fat diet.

When you are working out the rest of your body, you are exercising your heart as well. As you exercise more strenuously, your heart gets used to the increased demands placed upon it and learns to work harder as a result. Its size and strength increase. But the positive effects of training don't stop there. Your body's arteries and veins also benefit from having regular exercise. The number of capillaries in your heart increases, the amount of cholesterol deposits decreases, and cholesterol levels in your blood drop. If that's not enough, with low training zones your blood pressure will also drop.

The benefits of training don't stop even here. People who exercise regularly have a reduced risk of diabetes, obesity, osteoporosis, and some forms of cancer, and they almost always report an increase in energy and vitality. Regular exercise can decrease the incidence of depression, promote an overall reduction in stress, and enhance the flow of the natural chemicals that cause good feelings—like the "runner's high."

Even the spirit, some would argue, benefits from exercise. Professors at the Massachusetts Institute of Technology, Harvard, and Ohio State University have announced a relationship between exercise and feelings of spiritual peace and expansive oneness—the sort of condition more often connected with quiet meditation than a walk around the block. My own experience backs this up, and it isn't just that I run myself ragged, then bask in a glow of endorphins. Really, any time you set and follow through on a tangible goal, such as starting and continuing a fitness program, you are going to reap the benefits of increased confidence and contentment. The fact that your very body is changing, becoming better and stronger with training, is what makes reaching this particular goal so satisfying.

Deciding If Healthy Heart Zone Training Is Right for You

I recommend exclusive or predominant training in the Healthy Heart zone for two groups of people.

The first group is older adults like Roger. For out-of-shape folks in their fifties or sixties and in-shape people over seventy, the majority of workouts should be in the Healthy Heart zone. Working out more vigorously than this does not give more health benefits to this group; it only increases the risk of injury.

The second group is the 20 to 30 percent of the population who have known or suspected cardiovascular problems, like Margaret. For them, the Healthy Heart zone is ideal: It strengthens the heart safely. I can't tell you the number of people I've met who are in cardiac rehabilitation programs and who are training in the Healthy Heart zone on their cardiologists' recommendations. Cardiac rehabilitation always uses some form of exercise to improve a diseased heart. It has been repeatedly demonstrated that a moderate exercise program will reduce the risk of death from a subsequent heart attack and improve the quality of life for the patient.

The Healthy Heart Zone Training program may not be necessary for those who are merely overweight. If you are otherwise healthy, without any known or suspected cardiovascular problems, it is very likely you can start right in with the Weight Management program (see Chapter 4).

Before we jump ahead, though, let's walk through the preliminary steps to starting a Healthy Heart Zone Training program.

Step 1: Deciding Whether You Need a Medical Clearance

Your first level of pre-exercise screening is the Physical Activity Readiness Questionnaire (PAR-Q) that you answered on page 19 in Chapter 1. Those who are older or who have known health concerns might want to consider a few other factors. If you answer "yes" to any of the following questions, you should see your doctor.

1. Are you over 60 years old and unaccustomed to moderate exercise?
2. Does premature (before age 55) coronary artery disease run in your family?
3. After exercising, do you suffer from pain or feel pressure in the left side or middle of your chest, or in the left side of your neck, shoulder, or arm?
4. Have you felt faint or suffered severe dizziness after mild exercise?

5. Do you not know whether your blood pressure is normal or elevated, or has your doctor told you that your blood pressure is too high and uncontrolled?
6. Has your doctor told you that you have a heart problem, such as angina, arrhythmia, or a severe heart murmur?
7. Have you had a heart attack?
8. Have you experienced bone or joint problems such as arthritis?
9. Do you have any other medical conditions that might require additional attention if you began an exercise program?

Adapted from the U.S. National Heart, Lung, and Blood Institute (1981).

Margaret, age fifty-two, answered yes only to question 7, but that would have been enough to send her to the doctor's for a consultation and check-up if she had not already been under his supervision. Roger, at seventy-six, had to answer yes to question 1, and also to question 8, since he does have osteoarthritis in his knees. To remember to ask about the arthritis, he took this questionnaire with him when he went to his doctor for approval.

Step 2: Knowing the Answers

You've passed the PAR-Q test and you've answered the questions in Step 1, and (if necessary), you have your doctor's approval in hand. You're ready to go, right? Not quite. Before you actually begin your Healthy Heart Zone Training, I'd like you to go over a few commonly asked questions. The answers will put your program in the proper perspective.

- Will I develop "athlete's heart" if I Heart Zone Train?

  Answer: Yes and no. The term "athlete's heart" was coined in the late nineteenth century by those who thought that exercise damaged the heart by enlarging and weakening it. Today the term refers to cardiac characteristics such as lower ambient and resting heart rates, increased stroke volume, and improved cardiac output. So using the modern definition the answer is, yes, you will have an athlete's heart, and that's a good thing.

- Can I start Heart Zone Training if I have a heart murmur?

  Answer: Yes, with a medical clearance. It used to be that you were automatically disqualified from exercise if you had this condition. Now it's known that a vast majority of heart murmurs, particularly in fit individuals, are entirely "innocent" and their presence does not indicate heart disease. For example, 80 percent of all runners have heart murmurs; it's a feature of their fitness and not indicative of disease. The same runners also have a high incidence of abnormal heart rhythms. *In the absence of other symptoms*, this is normal and does not indicate heart disease.

- Can I work out if I have high blood pressure?

  Answer: If your systolic blood pressure is over 160 or your diastolic blood pressure is over 90, or if you are on anti-hypertensive medication, you fall into the classification for major coronary risk factors and should check in with your physician before starting any exercise program. That being said, exercise is certainly one of the prescriptions for lowering your blood pressure. In fact, if you want to eliminate medication for hypertension or decrease your blood pressure, living the Heart Zone

Training lifestyle is one of the best ways to do it. Make sure you train predominantly in the lower zones, however, since training in the higher zones will not have as much effect on your blood pressure.

- Can I exercise if I am a heart patient?

  Answer: Yes—but there are special considerations, because for you training is a safety issue. (That's why using a heart rate monitor to record your heart rate accurately is so important.) First, always follow your physician's instructions and stay in communication with her or him about your exercise program. Second, if training for long periods is hard, break your workout into shorter periods, such as five to fifteen minutes each, and do several in one day. Third, spend more time in your warm-up and cool-down periods before and after exercise. Fourth, stay in the two lower zones as much as possible. Finally, if you want to lift weights to increase muscle strength, that's great, but make sure you use the "circuit" style of moving from station to station and increasing the number of repetitions while decreasing the amount of weight you lift.

- I've heard that you shouldn't exercise, because you only have so many heartbeats in a lifetime and exercising just uses them up faster. Is this true?

  Answer: No. Each heartbeat is precious, yet your lifetime supply is limitless. The heart doesn't wear out after a certain number of contractions; no muscle does. And besides, the more you exercise, the fewer times your heart will contract. That's part of the magic of fitness—exercise more and save more. The more you Heart Zone Train, the lower your resting heart rate. If you can lower your resting heart rate to 58 bpm, which is quite normal for fit folks, you will save six million heartbeats each year, or over 400 million heartbeats in an average lifetime.

	NON-EXERCISER'S HEART	HEART ZONE TRAINER'S HEART
BEATS PER MINUTE AT REST	72	58
BEATS PER HOUR	4,320	3,480
BEATS PER DAY	103,680	83,520
ADDITIONAL BEATS USED DURING EXERCISE*	0	936,000
TOTAL BEATS PER YEAR	37,843,200	31,420,800
BEATS SAVED PER YEAR		6,422,400
BEATS SAVED IN 70 YEARS		449,568,000

Based on four thirty-minute workouts a week in the Aerobic zone (150 bpm).

Step 3: Beginning Your Healthy Heart Training Program

Though no one knows all the exact causes of coronary heart disease, we do know what the major lifestyle or risk factors are. The more risk factors or nonhealthy lifestyle habits you develop, the higher your risk.

Here's a quick way to help you evaluate how healthy you and your heart are. This test is not designed to replace a physician's evaluation, but it does give you an idea of what parts of your lifestyle may be influencing your risk of developing heart disease. Take the test by adding up the points in the boxes that best describe your current status. The lower the score, the healthier your heart, and the better your chances of not getting heart disease.

Some of the boxes, such as those for **Exercise**, **Age**, and **Weight**, are pretty straightforward, while others deserve a little more explanation. For **Heredity**, count parents, brothers, and sisters who have had a heart attack. With **Tobacco Use**, if you inhale deeply and smoke a cigarette way down, add one point to your score. (Do not subtract because you think you do not inhale or smoke only a half inch on a cigarette.) Under **Exercise**, lower your score one point if you exercise regularly and frequently. Regarding **Cholesterol/Saturated Fat Intake**, if you have not had a blood test recently, then estimate honestly the percentage of solid fats you eat. (These are usually of animal origin—beef, lamb, pork, or the fat that comes from these animals in lard or milk products.) For **Blood Pressure**, if you have no recent reading but have passed an insurance or general medical examination, chances are you have a systolic blood pressure level of 140 or less. **Gender** takes into account the fact that men have from six to ten times more heart attacks than women of child-bearing age, although more and more women have become prone to heart disease as a result of lifestyle choices such as smoking.

Sally Edwards' Heart Zone Training

MEASURING YOUR RISK FOR HEART DISEASE: YOUR LIFESTYLE TEST*

AGE	10–20	21–30	31–40	41–50	51–60	61–70+
	1	2	3	4	6	8
EXERCISE	Intensive exertion at work and in recreation	Moderate exertion at work and in recreation	Sedentary at work and intense exertion in recreation	Sedentary at work and moderate exertion in recreation	Sedentary at work and light exertion in recreation	Complete lack of exercise
	1	2	3	5	6	8
HEREDITY	No known history of heart disease in family	One relative over 60 with cardiovascular disease	More than one relative over 60 with cardiovascular disease	One relative under 60 with cardiovascular disease	Two relatives under 60 with cardiovascular disease	Three or more relatives under 60 with cardiovascular disease
	1	2	3	4	5	7
WEIGHT	More than 5 lb. under standard weight	Between 5 lb. under or over standard weight	6 to 20 lb. over standard weight	21 to 35 lb. over standard weight	36 to 50 lb. over standard weight	More than 50 lb. over standard weight
	0	1	2	3	5	7
TOBACCO USE	Nonsmoker	Cigar or pipe smoker	Smokes 10 or less cigarettes daily	Smokes 20 cigarettes daily	Smokes 30 cigarettes daily	Smokes 40 or more cigarettes daily
	0	1	2	4	6	10
CHOLESTEROL OR FAT % IN DIET	Cholesterol below 180 mg/dl	Cholesterol between 181 and 205 mg/dl	Cholesterol between 206 and 230 mg/dl	Cholesterol between 231 and 255 mg/dl	Cholesterol between 256 and 280 mg/dl	Cholesterol between 281 and 300 mg/dl
	Diet with no animal or solid fats 1	Diet with 10% animal or solid fats 2	Diet with 20% animal or solid fats 3	Diet with 30% animal or solid fats 4	Diet with 40% animal or solid fats 5	Diet with 50% or more animal or solid fats 7
BLOOD PRESSURE	Upper reading between 100 and 119	Upper reading between 120 and 139	Upper reading between 140 and 159	Upper reading between 160 and 179	Upper reading between 180 and 199	Upper reading over 200
	1	2	3	4	6	8
GENDER	Female under 40 years old	Female between 40 and 50 years old	Female over 50 years old	Male	Stocky male	Bald stocky male
	1	2	3	4	6	7

*The Coronary Heart Disease Risk Appraisal (RISKO) adapted from the Michigan Heart Association.

After taking the test, score your results according to the following chart, then use your score to determine your specific Heart Zone Training recommendations.

SCORE	LEVEL OF RISK	HEART ZONE TRAINING RECOMMENDATIONS
6–11	Risk well below average	You are probably already on an exercise program—keep it up.
12–17	Risk below average	Begin your program today.
18–24	Average risk	Start slowly and progress.
25–31	Moderate risk	Stay in the Healthy Heart zone for at least the first month.
32–40	High risk	Stay in the Healthy Heart zone for the first two months and get a medical check-up.
41–62	Very high risk, see your physician	Don't begin until you have a clearance from your physician.

Here's how Margaret's and Roger's tests turned out:

Margaret

Age: fifty-two years old. **6 points**.

Exercise: Margaret not only hasn't exercised for years, as an office manager she sits all day at work, so she had to choose "Complete lack of exercise." **8 points**.

Heredity: Margaret's father had a heart attack at age sixty-eight. **2 points**.

Weight: Margaret's doctor has warned her that she is about forty pounds overweight. **5 points**.

Tobacco Use: Margaret smokes about a half pack a day, although she is trying very hard to cut down. **2 points**.

Cholesterol: Margaret's cholesterol level is 246. **4 points**.

Blood Pressure: Margaret's systolic blood pressure is currently 143, although she and her physician are working to lower it. **3 points**.

Gender: Margaret is a female over fifty. **3 points**.

This makes Margaret's total *33 points*, placing her at high risk for recurrence of heart problems. The test brought home to Margaret that cutting down on her smoking, losing some weight, and starting an exercise program really would lower her chances of further heart disease. She decided to post the test on her fridge at home as a reminder.

Roger

Age: seventy-six years old. **8 points**.

Exercise: Roger figured that his writing was his work, now that he's retired, and the golf, fishing, and gold panning counted as some form of exercise, so he selected "Sedentary work and light recreational exertion." **6 points**.

Heredity: Roger has no known history of heart disease in his family. **1 point**.

Weight: Roger is about fifteen pounds overweight. **2 points**.

Tobacco Use: Roger loves the occasional cigar. **1 point**.

Cholesterol: Roger's cholesterol is 212. He has a daughter who is a vegetarian and has been trying to get him to cut down on the amount of meat he eats, but she hasn't had much luck yet. Now that he's taken this test, Roger thinks maybe he'll give her veggie burgers one more try. **3 points**.

Blood Pressure: Roger's systolic blood pressure is 117. **1 point**.

Gender: Roger is a tall, moderate-built male. **4 points**.

Roger's total is **26 points**, putting him at moderate risk of heart disease. He was a little frustrated that he earned 12 of his 26 points just by being an older male, but he reasoned that he could still do a lot to help himself by starting to exercise more regularly and by cutting down on his beloved cigars and pork chops.

If your score is high now, challenge yourself to lower it.

How? We do know what one of the major risk *decreasers* is **exercise**. You may have been born with a healthy heart, but as you grow older, you have to work at it. You can't just eat a low-fat diet and get a healthy heart. You can't just quit smoking or start a stress-reduction class, either. Having a healthy heart is the sum of lifestyle changes, first and foremost among which should be regular exercise.

Getting a Healthier Heart: The Healthy Heart Zone Program

At 50 to 60 percent of your Max HR, the Healthy Heart zone is the easiest of the five Heart Zone Training zones to work out in. It's ideal for beginners and those with special needs because it's fun, it's comfortable, and it creates cardiovascular benefits while burning some fat and giving you a clear sense of accomplishment. For me, this zone is 100 to 120 bpm (50 percent to 60 percent of my Max HR of 200 bpm). Determine the range of your Healthy Heart zone from the chart below and use it to fill in the floor and ceiling number for your Healthy Heart Zone Training program.

MAXIMUM HEART RATE AND THE HEALTHY HEART ZONE

MAX HR	155	160	165	170	175	180	185	190	195	200	205	210
50% (floor)	78	80	83	85	88	90	93	95	98	100	103	105
60% (ceiling)	93	96	99	102	105	108	111	114	117	120	123	126

Before we start into the program, I want to remind you once again: Don't overdo it. Why? Because overdoing it isn't necessary, for starters. You *will* get a noticeable benefit just from three or four brief Healthy Heart zone workouts each week. Overdoing it can actually keep you from gaining the very benefits you seek. Remember the story of my brother Chris? He wasn't able to go off his blood pressure medication until he slowed himself down, dropping out of the Aerobic zone and doing Healthy Heart zone workouts instead.

In Chapter 2 we put together an initial thirty-day program. For the Healthy Heart zone program, we're talking in terms of *months*, not weeks. For people like Margaret, Roger, and you, short-term athletic improvement is not the issue; long-term health results are. Healthy heart results start immediately upon beginning the program, but they accumulate over a long period of time, and those with special needs should focus on safety, first and foremost. To play it safe with any exercise program, make changes gradually.

If, after a month, you feel ready to increase your efforts, move ahead to the next month of the program; then, at the end of the second month, move ahead to the third. Resist the impulse to push yourself ahead faster than that. You've got plenty of time to get fit, so why not take it? By the same token, if you don't feel ready to move ahead at any time, don't. It's that simple. *Continue* with the first month's basic Healthy Heart zone program, however, as long as your physician thinks it's advisable.

Be sure to monitor your heart rate during your Healthy Heart zone workouts. It's very easy to push yourself too hard; one slight uphill on an otherwise flat walk can raise your heart rate by 10 to 30 bpm. You are focusing on one thing and one thing only here: the Healthy Heart zone. Take advantage of the repeated workouts and really get to know the zone. Once you are used to your normal pace for the various activities you do in the Healthy Heart zone, you'll be surprised what will influence your heart rates. A head cold, a bad mood, or an especially warm or cold day will probably throw your heart rate and pacing off. For that matter, so will dehydration. This is less of a factor at lower heart rates, but you should still remember to drink plenty of fluids before, during, and after exercising.

Month 1

Margaret and Roger were both starting pretty much from scratch with their programs, so their doctors advised them to begin with very light and brief workout sessions. Margaret wasn't sure what form of exercise she'd like best, so she "shopped around" during her first month and tried various alternatives. Her first month's plan looked like this:

MARGARET MONTH 1	SUNDAY	MONDAY	TUESDAY	WEDNESDAY	THURSDAY	FRIDAY	SATURDAY	WEEKLY SUMMARY
ACTIVITY	Rest	Walk	Rest	Swim	Rest	Circuit Train	Bike	4 activities
FREQUENCY		1		1		1	1	4 workouts
INTENSITY		Healthy Heart		Healthy Heart		Healthy Heart	Healthy Heart	1 zone
TIME		15 minutes		15 minutes		15 minutes	15 minutes	60 minutes

At first Margaret wasn't sure whether she wanted to work out three days per week or four. She started out just exercising for fifteen minutes before work on Monday, Wednesday, and Friday, but after two weeks her husband asked to join in on the weekends, so now they go for a leisurely bike ride together at a local park, bringing Margaret's exercise schedule up to four times a week. Margaret likes the fifteen-minute length of her sessions, since any more than that tends to make her feel tired. By the end of the month her cardiologist reported that her cholesterol level had dropped by five points, and she saw by her bathroom scale that she'd lost three pounds.

Roger is of the no-time-like-the-present, get-up-and-get-to-it school, and his first month's log reflected this:

ROGER MONTH 1	SUNDAY	MONDAY	TUESDAY	WEDNESDAY	THURSDAY	FRIDAY	SATURDAY	WEEKLY SUMMARY
ACTIVITY	Rest	Walk	Walk	Rest	Walk	Walk	Rest	1 activity
FREQUENCY		1	1		1	1		4 workouts
INTENSITY		Healthy Heart	Healthy Heart		Healthy Heart	Healthy Heart		1 zone
TIME		20 minutes	20 minutes		20 minutes	20 minutes		80 minutes

Through the local senior citizens' center Roger heard about group walks that other older gentlemen were taking each day. He decided to take part in the beginner's group sessions for twenty minutes a day, four mornings a week, strolling around town with a few companions. Roger kept to his schedule, even when it rained; then the group met for their walk inside the local shopping mall. Roger found the walks to be a convenient and social activity, and he's already lost five pounds! He called his doctor to report the results because he was actually a little worried about losing weight so quickly. He was told that all sounded well and that he should expect his weight to stabilize after the first couple of months. Roger liked the fact that he was able to make a weekly workout schedule that kept his weekends free for his drives into the Sierra and other recreational activities.

Month 2

By the second month most folks are eager to try adding a little more time to their schedule. Margaret and her doctor came to the conclusion that she could add slightly to her workouts over the next month, if she wished. Her log for the month looked like this:

MARGARET MONTH 2	SUNDAY	MONDAY	TUESDAY	WEDNESDAY	THURSDAY	FRIDAY	SATURDAY	WEEKLY SUMMARY
ACTIVITY	Rest	Walk	Rest	Floor Exercises	Rest	Circuit Train	Bike	4 activities
FREQUENCY		1		1		1	1	4 workouts
INTENSITY		Healthy Heart		Healthy Heart		Healthy Heart	Healthy Heart	1 zone
TIME		15 minutes		20 minutes		15 minutes	20 minutes	70 minutes

Margaret decided to add five minutes to her bike rides, since her husband was eager to go a little further and she found the rides pretty non-wearing. She also wanted an alternative to her swim sessions, since she realized she was coming to hate the whole process of showering and doing her hair twice on Wednesdays. As an alternative she picked up the twenty-minute floor portion of a morning exercise class at her gym. She likes the fact that she's toning up while in a comfortable social setting. All in all, Margaret added ten minutes to her total workout time each week, enough to make it interesting and increase her fitness benefits, but not so much as to put her at any risk of injury. And at the end of the month, her doctor's scale revealed that she had lost another three pounds.

Roger has found that all the walking makes his knees hurt, so he wants to adapt his schedule a little to compensate for that. His Month 2 log looks like this:

ROGER MONTH 2	SUNDAY	MONDAY	TUESDAY	WEDNESDAY	THURSDAY	FRIDAY	SATURDAY	WEEKLY SUMMARY
ACTIVITY	Rest	Walk	Swim	Rest	Walk	Swim	Rest	2 activities
FREQUENCY		1	1		1	1		4 workouts
INTENSITY		Healthy Heart	Healthy Heart		Healthy Heart	Healthy Heart		1 zone
TIME		20 minutes	30 minutes		20 minutes	30 minutes		100 minutes

Roger's doctor recommended switching half his walking workouts for swims for a month, to see whether that helped his knees. That was fine by Roger, who still gets to visit with his walking group two days a week and is now making new acquaintances at the local public pool, during their senior swim periods. Since he likes to swim at a leisurely pace, he's comfortable spending a little more time in the water than he was doing pounding the pavement, so he has ended up adding twenty minutes to his weekly workout time. At the end of the month Roger's doctor told him that his cholesterol was down by six points so far. Roger had also lost another two pounds. He thought that was remarkable, but his daughter suggested that since he had always been quite slim, even underweight as a younger man, that perhaps with a little exercise his body was just getting back into its proper balance and adding muscle weight.

Month 3

During the third month you may gradually wish to increase your times-in-zone, or perhaps your workout frequency. Be aware that whenever you increase the duration of a session, you increase the likelihood that by the end of the session your heart rates may have drifted slightly upward out of the Healthy Heart zone. Keep checking your monitor or taking your pulse regularly, and you should be able to adjust your pace as needed.

Margaret's Month 3 log reflects her growing energy and enthusiasm for working out:

MARGARET MONTH 3	SUNDAY	MONDAY	TUESDAY	WEDNESDAY	THURSDAY	FRIDAY	SATURDAY	WEEKLY SUMMARY
ACTIVITY	Walk	Bike	Rest	Floor Exercises	Rest	Circuit Train	Bike	4 activities
FREQUENCY	1	1		1		1	1	5 workouts
INTENSITY	Healthy Heart	Healthy Heart		Healthy Heart		Healthy Heart	Healthy Heart	1 zone
TIME	20 minutes	20 minutes		20 minutes		15 minutes	20 minutes	95 minutes

Actually, Margaret isn't the only one with newfound enthusiasm for exercise. She added her Sunday walk at her husband's request! They both enjoyed the carefree time they spent together on their bike rides, and he wanted more. This change allowed Margaret to rethink the rest of her schedule, and she decided that she liked cycling so much she wanted to do it Mondays, too, on the stationary bike at the gym. Because she and her husband liked slightly longer workouts together, and because she had been getting fitter all this time, Margaret was able to add five minutes to her walk times for a total of twenty minutes. She made her stationary bike workouts twenty minutes long too, because that was what she was used to. All in all she added twenty-five minutes added to her weekly times. Again, not too much, not too little.

Margaret has yet to be bored with her new routine and is very pleased with her overall results. With the additional workout she has lost four pounds this month, bringing her total loss to ten pounds of excess weight at the end of three months on her Healthy Heart Zone Training program. Her doctor's tests have confirmed that her cholesterol levels dropped from 246 to 234 over this period, a difference of twelve points. Margaret is also reporting an increase in her energy level and a great lessening of the sadness and anxiety she had felt after her heart attack. She and her doctor agree that further gradual increases in her exercise frequency, time, and, eventually, intensity are the way to go.

Roger has been delighted with his newfound vim and vigor, and with his doctor's approval decides to add a bit more time to his weekly schedule. His Month 3 log reflects this:

ROGER MONTH 3	SUNDAY	MONDAY	TUESDAY	WEDNESDAY	THURSDAY	FRIDAY	SATURDAY	WEEKLY SUMMARY
ACTIVITY	Rest	Walk	Swim	Rest	Walk	Swim	Rest	2 activities
FREQUENCY		1	1		1	1		4 workouts
INTENSITY		Healthy Heart	Healthy Heart		Healthy Heart	Healthy Heart		1 zone
TIME		30 minutes	30 minutes		30 minutes	30 minutes		120 minutes

Roger decided it might be time to try joining the intermediate group of walkers, who go on slightly longer walks. By the end of the month, though, his knees were hurting him again, and he was missing his beginner walking group buddies, so he decided to switch back. A trip to his doctor's office confirmed a total decrease over the three months of eight points on his cholesterol levels, from 212 to 204, as well as the loss of another three pounds, bringing his total weight loss to eleven pounds. Roger celebrated by going out for a trip with his daughter to buy some better walking shoes! Roger and his doctor agree that no further increases in frequency, time, or intensity will be necessary. So long as Roger keeps to his current schedule, he should be doing very well for some time to come.

At the end of the three months, if you and your physician agree that an increase in your FIT (frequency, intensity, and time) is a good idea, try moving into the beginning of the Weight Management program (see Chapter 4). Even if you don't need to lose any weight, working out in the Temperate zone will keep your weight stable and give you further cardiovascular benefits, along with a little more of a challenge.

Healthy Heart Zone Activities

Take the activities suggested below as just that: suggestions. As long as you keep your heart rate within the Healthy Heart zone, anything goes!

Walking

WORKOUT	ACTIVITY
Hills	Find a rolling course that has at least one- to two-minute elevation changes. Walk hard on the uphills, so that you hit the top or ceiling of your zone, and go easy on the downhills, so that your heart rate drops back down to the bottom or floor again before you ascend another hill.

Steady-State | Pick a specific heart rate in the middle of your Healthy Heart zone and walk the entire time as close as possible to that specific heart rate number.

Partner | Take a friend with you on your usual walk. You will notice that when you walk and talk, your heart rate goes up about five beats from the heart rate required to walk the route alone.

Maximum Steady-State | This is like the steady-state walk, but this time you aim for the top number of your Healthy Heart zone and walk at this heart rate throughout the walk.

Bicycling

WORKOUT	ACTIVITY
Hills	Cycling hills, whether outdoors or on an indoor stationary bike, can be fun, because it gives you a change in effort or workload. It's also challenging, because you'll have to go easy on the uphills and hard on the downhills to stay within the top and bottom limits of your heart rate zone.
Steady-State	Pick a specific heart rate in the middle of your Healthy Heart zone and work out the entire time at that heart rate number. Keep in mind that if you get tired, your heart rate may go up, and you may have to slow down to compensate.
Maximum Steady-State	Exercise the whole time at the top heart rate in your Healthy Heart zone.

Swimming

WORKOUT	ACTIVITY
Criss-Cross	Swim the length of the pool without stopping. If you aren't too tired by that, try swimming out and back without stopping (one lap). In between lengths or laps, rest. This is a criss-cross workout; that means you will criss-cross the Healthy Heart zone. When you are swimming, aim for a heart rate number at the top of your zone; then rest until your heart rate drops down to the floor of the zone again. Then push off from the wall again.
Midpoint Steady-State	This is one long, slow, steady, continuous swim for the entire period of time. Pick the midpoint in your zone and hold it for the entire swim without stopping. If you like to stop, then swim for five minutes at a time, with a thirty-second rest in between to get your heart rate down.
Training Toys	They are actually called "training devices," and all swimmers use them: fins, buoys, tubes, kick boards, hand paddles, etc. They help you isolate a part of your body and work on strengthening it. Most pools provide them at no cost. Pick out three of your favorites and swim for five minutes with each swim toy, changing at the end of each five-minute period and making sure you always stay in your Healthy Heart zone.

Fitness Classes/Equipment

WORKOUT	ACTIVITY
Aerobics Class	Either buy a video tape or go to a club and join an aerobics class. Tell your instructor that you are doing Heart Zone Training and would like to zone train in his or her class, which means you will be adjusting your movements to stay within your Healthy Heart zone. Do the entire class, but monitor your heart rate every couple of minutes and adjust your movements so that you stay within your zone. Your instructor should be able to help you.
Cardio-Circuit Training	When you do circuit training at a fitness center, you can bounce around from one cardiovascular machine to the next, never getting bored. Pick out four of your favorite pieces, like the treadmill, exercise bike, rowing machine, and stairstepper, and stay with each for five minutes, then rotate to the next without a break.
Weight Training	This is like circuit training, but you stay within your zones as you move from weight station to weight station. Include both your upper body and lower body muscle groups as you circuit the stations.

Basketball

WORKOUT	ACTIVITY
Intervals	The fun of shooting interval hoops is that you are rewarded for hitting the basket. Every time you miss you have to jog or walk to half- or full-court

	and back before you shoot again. If you sink the ball, you get to keep shooting until you miss.
Steady-State Lay-Ups	Without leaving your Healthy Heart zone, dribble your way from one end of the court to the other, shooting lay-ups. (For you novices that means that when you reach the basket, you bounce the ball off the glass and through the hoop.) It's a good time to practice your left-hand (nondominant) dribbling.
Half-Court One-on-One	It's not easy to stay in a low zone playing this way, but it's really fun if you have a heart rate monitor with an alarm that goes off if you go outside the zone. The opposing player gets a free-throw shot each time the other player's alarm goes off. It teaches you to keep consciously relaxed!
Playing the Game	Coaches like to call it "going at 75 percent," as opposed to full-out. It's best to play half-court, but set your zones and listen for the alarm, if your monitor has one. If things get too intense, have everyone agree to go at "60 percent." As the game slows down, dribbling and passing skills will probably improve.

Your Personal Log

Unlike the log at the end of Chapter 2, this one covers a three-month period. Don't fill it all out at once. Like Margaret and Roger, you should adapt each successive month's activities and the FIT for those activities as you learn more about your own needs and preferences. These logs should record not only what you plan to do but what you actually have done.

Sally Edwards' Heart Zone Training

HEART ZONE TRAINING LOG

	SUNDAY	MONDAY	TUESDAY	WEDNESDAY	THURSDAY	FRIDAY	SATURDAY	WEEKLY SUMMARY
ACTIVITY								
FREQUENCY								
INTENSITY								
TIME								

Managing Your Weight 4

On a flight to Boston last year I sat next to a young man named Brad. Brad was about sixty pounds overweight. When he saw that I ate only the salad off my dinner tray, he asked if he could have my cellophane-wrapped dessert cake. Between mouthfuls he confessed, "I know I eat too much. Working at a desk in front of a computer all day, I've gained a lot of weight since I got out of college three years ago. I tried counting calories, but figuring out just how much I could eat of every little thing was a real pain and didn't make me any less hungry. I know I should exercise, too, but that has always bored me to death. I've tried six different diet plans, but I've always come back to the see-food diet: When I see food, I eat it."

I happened to be working on this book during the flight, writing a chapter on my laptop, and as usual I was wearing my heart rate monitor. Brad was fascinated by the technology. He asked for information on how he could buy one and use it to manage his weight. A month later he sent me this note:

"I bought a basic heart rate monitor, Sally, along with your book. The whole idea of getting immediate feedback on my heart rate and using it to lose weight really appealed to me. I decided I have nothing to lose but my fat, so I'm starting the Temperate zone program today."

Marcia, the veterinarian who cares for my Australian cattle dog, Allez Allez, made it to age forty-one before ever having to worry about her weight. She attributes this to the fact that she's always moving at work and has generally eaten wisely over the years, but over the past year or two she's gained ten pounds and, as she puts it, "They're all in the wrong places!" Now forty-three, Marcia wants a moderate-intensity exercise plan that will help her lose those few extra pounds and keep them off without taking up too much of her scarce time and energy. On my recommendation, she's started a Heart Zone weight management program too. Keep reading to learn how Brad and Marcia managed their weight with Heart Zone Training.

The Fat-Burning Side of Temperate Zone

Folks who are already in great shape need not worry about what kind of calories they burn, but if, like the majority of the population, you want to lose weight or just keep from gaining weight, you may want to join Brad and Marcia in a program that will ensure that you are working off fat calories in the most efficient way possible. Heart Zone Training in the Temperate zone does just that.

Exercising in the Temperate zone allows you to burn excess body fat—how much depends on the exercise intensity, the amount of excess fat you have, your nutritional habits, the food you just ate, the activities you do, your frame size, your genetics, your basal metabolic rate, and your lean or muscle weight. In other words, it's complicated.

In the Temperate zone, about 85 percent of all the calories you burn come from dietary fat and your fat stores. Whereas you can expect to burn roughly six calories per minute in the Healthy Heart zone, in the Temperate zone you can burn as many as ten. In other words, during ten minutes of exercise in that zone, depending on your weight and other factors, you could burn as much as one hundred calories, including eighty-five from fat—again depending on a number of factors. As you continue to train into the higher zones, you may burn more calories, but you will be burning more carbohydrate calories. Consider the following chart:

ZONE	% OF MAX HR	ENERGY EXPANDED	FUELS BURNED (APPROX.)
Healthy Heart Zone	50–60% Max HR	4–6 calories per minute	85% Fat 10% Carbohydrate 5% Protein
Temperate Zone	60–70% Max HR	6–10 calories per minute	70% Fat 25% Carbohydrate 5% Protein
Aerobic Zone	70–80% Max HR	10–12 calories per minute	35% Fat 60% Carbohydrate 5% Protein

Workouts in the Temperate zone involve a moderate level of activity, not strenuous but challenging, where you feel the effects of your exercise. You break a sweat, but you can still carry on a conversation the entire time without feeling any discomfort. Once you go beyond this zone, you'll notice the difference in your effort and heart rate, because in zones higher than Temperate zone intensities you'll be gaining more in terms of fitness than health.

When you exercise in the Temperate zone, you double your health rewards, disposing of body fat while gaining muscle mass. The more muscle mass you develop, the more you can burn fat calories while just sitting still.

Once you get into relatively good shape, you can hang out in the Temperate zone for longer periods of time, using it as a recovery zone after heavier workouts or as a long endurance zone. If you use the Temperate zone for endurance, the blend of fuels your body burns becomes even more favorable. With longer training sessions your body begins to run out of the readily available carbohydrates in your system and begins drawing more heavily from your body's fat stores. The longer the exercise duration, the more body fat you consume, or metabolize. That's what's so great about long, slow training—it increases your "fat mobilization."

A word of caution, however: Don't expect to start a Heart Zone Training program and see big improvements on your second day. When you add a weight-management component to your training, you won't lose weight immediately, nor will you trim inches from your figure. It takes time. Don't think you can "beat the system." You can't. Heart Zone Training works *with* the system, taking advantage of how the body works; it doesn't produce results overnight.

If you've set weight management as a goal, don't feel alone. Young or old, rich or poor, most of us put on too much weight. Even kids have this problem nowadays. According to a 1995 National Health and Nutrition Examination Survey by the National Center for Health Statistics, kids have been getting fatter and fatter every year for the past thirty years. They've been gaining excess weight for the same reasons their parents have—a combination of inactivity and high-calorie foods. Thanks to personal computers and video games, a lot of kids (and adults) are building well-developed fingers and wrists, but not much else!

My experience with the children of my family and friends has shown me that exercising using Heart Zone Training and a heart rate monitor can give kids all the technological kicks they want. Some sophisticated heart rate monitors allow you to download information into your computer, adding a fascinating dimension to Heart Zone Training. Kids can have fun using their computers and their heart rate monitors to win the fight against childhood obesity.

The Temperate Zone Training Program

People who exercise for weight loss benefit from setting specific goals. Goals help gauge progress.

Brad's goals looked like this:

1. Within two months, be able to walk a mile in twenty minutes.
2. Eat only my allotted number of grams of fat every day; log both my time-in-zone and my daily fat grams for two months.
3. Reduce my weight by the end of two months.

   Marcia's goals looked like this:

1. Add one workout to my weekly schedule.

2. Firm up or get more muscle tone within one month, increase lean or muscle mass, and decrease percentage of body fat.
3. Maintain or slightly decrease my total body weight by the end of one month.

Set no more than three goals, and keep them reasonable. Note that neither Brad nor Marcia included anything along the lines of "lose twenty pounds by next month." That kind of goal can be a recipe for frustration and failure. Your body will lose as much weight as it loses. Trying to force a certain amount of weight loss in a certain amount of time almost always results in the dreaded "weight bounce-back." Remember, in Heart Zone Training you are striving for gradual, permanent changes in your body and your lifestyle, not some overnight miracle. The best results come from taking it slow and easy.

Whatever your own personal goals, write them down and post them in a highly visible place where you will see them every day. Brad kept his weight management program and goals posted on his computer's screen saver; Marcia taped hers to the bathroom mirror at home and at the clinic.

Remember, once you have identified your Max HR, you can set your Temperate zone yourself by calculating 60 to 70 percent of your Max HR, or you can take the values from the table below. Either way, make sure you determine the floor and ceiling for your particular zone.

MAXIMUM HEART RATE AND THE TEMPERATE ZONE

MAX HR	155	160	165	170	175	180	185	190	195	200	205	210
60% (floor)	93	96	99	102	105	108	111	114	117	120	123	126
70% (ceiling)	109	112	116	119	123	126	130	133	137	140	144	147

Once you've set your personal 60 to 70 percent zone, you can, like Brad and Marcia, design your own specific weight management program.

Week 1

Approaching his first week, Brad felt a little uncertain about what activity to choose. Having not exercised regularly since childhood, and not having been very active even then, he wasn't sure what he'd be good at or even enjoy. We talked about whether he could walk or cycle to and from work, but that turned out to be impossible, since he lives about twenty miles from his workplace. He also said he did not want to get up early in order to exercise, because he already gets up quite early enough to avoid heavy traffic. On top of that, because Brad admits to being a bit of a workaholic (a tendency related to his obesity), he usually works about eleven or twelve hours a day and so doesn't get home until 8:00 or 9:00 P.M., at which point he eats and gets into bed to read or watch TV. These are not great lifestyle habits and lead to self-defeating behaviors. I told Brad I was amazed he wasn't more overweight, and suggested he use his lunch hour to exercise. He reluctantly admitted that his company, a large computer firm, maintained a gym on the premises and that it wouldn't cost him anything to use it.

I reminded Brad that what activity he chose didn't matter so much as the zone in which he performed that activity, and that as long as he remembered to check his heart rate frequently, he could be doing anything he liked. He had planned simply to start out with fifteen minutes a day in the Temperate zone on Monday, Wednesday, and Friday. His actual schedule, however, turned out like this:

Sally Edwards' Heart Zone Training

BRAD WEEK 1	SUNDAY	MONDAY	TUESDAY	WEDNESDAY	THURSDAY	FRIDAY	SATURDAY	WEEKLY SUMMARY
ACTIVITY	Rest	Stair Step	Cycle	Rest	Rest	Treadmill	Rest	3 activities
FREQUENCY		1	1			1		3 workouts
INTENSITY		Temperate	Temperate			Temperate (20 minutes) Aerobic (10 minutes)		2 zones
TIME		15 minutes	20 minutes			30 minutes		65 minutes

When Brad finally visited the gym on Monday, he quickly discovered lots of interesting (from his engineer's perspective) machines. He used the stair-stepper on Monday at lunch and felt great the rest of the afternoon. On Tuesday he decided to use one of the electronic cycles, and losing track of time, he pedaled for twenty minutes. On Friday he woke up and went to work and all he could think about was trying out another piece of workout equipment. That day he went to lunch early and ended up so fascinated by the treadmill that he really got carried away with adjusting its elevation and speed, and he ended up doing a thirty-minute workout that took him well up into his Aerobic zone before he finished. Not surprisingly, Brad said he felt good Friday afternoon but somewhat worn out over the weekend. When Monday rolled around again, however, he felt motivated and energized to resume his weekly program.

Before starting the weight management program, Brad had checked with his doctor, who measured his current percentage of body fat and gave him a green light to start a low-intensity exercise routine. He had also put his Heart Zone Training log on his computer and started recording his plan and workouts. When we reviewed his first week, Brad agreed that he hadn't seen any dramatic results as far as weight loss went, but he felt good about his program. The fun "toys," as he put it, had kept the exercise from being boring, and the schedule we had set up had worked well. I told him he should consider his first week a resounding success.

Marcia started out with a different set of problems from Brad's. She worried that if she tried to exercise during the day, one or another of the usual office emergencies would cause her to miss her schedule more often than not. We therefore decided that she should consider an early-morning, prework exercise agenda. Marcia decided on a jog through a nearby park for her morning workout: "It's a beautiful area, and I always wish I could spend more time there. I often see my animal patients and their owners, and it's a lot of fun for all of us to socialize outside the office!" Marcia's Week 1 program ended up looking like this:

MARCIA WEEK 1	SUNDAY	MONDAY	TUESDAY	WEDNESDAY	THURSDAY	FRIDAY	SATURDAY	WEEKLY SUMMARY
ACTIVITY	Rest	Jog	Rest	Jog	Rest	Jog	Rest	1 activity
FREQUENCY		1		1		1		3 workouts
INTENSITY		Temperate		Temperate		Temperate		1 zone
TIME		20 minutes		20 minutes		20 minutes		60 minutes

At the end of the week, Marcia said she had found it easier than she expected to add the workouts to her schedule. Always a morning person, she usually did paperwork or read before going to work; now she pulls on a pair of sweats and goes for a jog-walk. She said the intensity seemed to be just right—she never found her energy lagging later in the day from having worked herself too hard—and the frequency seemed right, too, although she had begun considering another, more strenuous jog on Sunday.

Week 2

For Brad, Week 2 became a chance to show that he understood and could stick to his schedule now. He did say that he'd like to increase his frequency to four times a week so that he could include a day of circuit training in the Healthy Heart zone, and I told him that sounded fine, as long as he remembered to keep closer track of his time-in-zone and of his intensities. I suggested that setting the alarm on his heart rate monitor to go off when his heart rate went over 130 bpm, the top of his Temperate zone, would remind him to slow himself down whenever necessary. Here's how Brad's Week 2 program worked out:

BRAD WEEK 2	SUNDAY	MONDAY	TUESDAY	WEDNESDAY	THURSDAY	FRIDAY	SATURDAY	WEEKLY SUMMARY
ACTIVITY	Rest	Stair Step	Rest	Cycle	Treadmill	Circuit Train	Rest	4 activities
FREQUENCY		1		1	1	1		4 workouts
INTENSITY		Temperate		Temperate	Temperate	Temperate		1 zone
TIME		15 minutes		15 minutes	15 minutes	15 minutes		60 minutes

Brad was true to his word, performing his scheduled workouts during Week 2 exactly as planned. He set the alarm on his heart rate monitor to go off both when his heart beat too fast and when it beat too slow for his chosen zone. He also found that working out three days in a row was fine, since he took two days of rest afterward. Brad also said that he's been noticing that since he started working out, he's lost the craving for his usual afternoon pick-me-ups: chocolate candy bars. So far, so good.

For Week 2, Marcia decided she'd like to add a weekend workout to her exercise schedule, although she worried a bit about wearing herself out with exercise. I suggested that since she was already doing three Temperate zone workouts to meet her weight management goals, that maybe she should consider doing a lower-intensity, Healthy Heart workout on the weekend rather than a more strenuous one. That appealed to her, so she settled on a leisurely Sunday bike ride as her fourth workout. Marcia's final Week 2 schedule turned out like this:

MARCIA WEEK 2	SUNDAY	MONDAY	TUESDAY	WEDNESDAY	THURSDAY	FRIDAY	SATURDAY	WEEKLY SUMMARY
ACTIVITY	Bike	Jog	Rest	Jog	Rest	Jog	Rest	2 activities
FREQUENCY	1	1		1		1		4 workouts
INTENSITY	Healthy Heart	Temperate		Temperate		Temperate		2 zones
TIME	35 minutes	20 minutes		20 minutes		20 minutes		95 minutes

After Week 2 Marcia said she'd begun to forget that she had ever run out of energy during the day. Each of her workouts made her feel healthier and more energized than she had in years. "I'm always telling my clients about how important it is to exercise their pets—maybe I should be telling them to exercise themselves, while they're at it!"

Marcia also felt really happy about how well her bike ride had turned out. "It was the perfect amount of unhurried exertion. I stayed in my Healthy Heart zone while cruising the neighborhood on my bike. I'm going to get a friend to come with me next week!"

Week 3

By Week 3 Brad toyed with the idea of spending a little more time with each workout, but he knew that he shouldn't add too much time, or he might risk overdoing it. He didn't want discomfort to harm his motivation. In fact, he was already growing bored with the cycling. He decided to add another treadmill session, which he enjoyed immensely. He could measure his progress by tracking his mileage and calories consumed, and the workout gave him a chance to listen to jazz on his cassette headphones. Brad's Week 3 looked like this:

BRAD WEEK 3	SUNDAY	MONDAY	TUESDAY	WEDNESDAY	THURSDAY	FRIDAY	SATURDAY	WEEKLY SUMMARY
ACTIVITY	Rest	Treadmill	Stair Step	Rest	Treadmill	Circuit Train	Rest	3 activities
FREQUENCY		1	1		1	1		4 workouts
INTENSITY		Temperate	Temperate		Temperate	Temperate		1 zone
TIME		20 minutes	20 minutes		20 minutes	20 minutes		80 minutes

This week finds his energy way up over what it was just three weeks ago, and he not only no longer craves chocolate bars in the afternoon, when a coworker offers him one, he opts for a banana and an apple instead. When he can no longer resist climbing onto his bathroom scale, he finds that he has lost three pounds. That may not seem like much, but his clothes fit a little more loosely. Wisely, however, he decides to hold off celebrating until after he visits his doctor for a quick check-up at the end of the month, during which he will have his fat percent measured again.

For Marcia, Week 3 brought frustration, then a few surprises. Her week started with a cold rain, canceling her Sunday bike ride and her Monday jog. When Tuesday morning dawned stormy again, Marcia decided enough was enough, packed up her gym bag, and drove downtown to a gym. She paid a one-day entry fee, then stepped into the beginning of a low-impact aerobics class, where she took care not to work herself so hard that her heart rate would zoom out of the Temperate zone. Her Week 3 weight management plan schedule ended up looking like this:

MARCIA WEEK 3	SUNDAY	MONDAY	TUESDAY	WEDNESDAY	THURSDAY	FRIDAY	SATURDAY	WEEKLY SUMMARY
ACTIVITY	Rest	Rest	Aerobics	Jog	Rest	Jog	Rest	2 activities
FREQUENCY			1	1		1		3 workouts
INTENSITY			Temperate	Temperate		Temperate		1 zone
TIME			20 minutes	20 minutes		20 minutes		60 minutes

When we talked after Week 3, Marcia reported really enjoying her week's workouts, especially the aerobics class in the club. "It's so motivating to be around all these other people who are working out too," she said. "I don't feel bad about missing my bike ride or Monday's jog, because Week 3 taught me two things: First, even with the best of intentions, you can't always stick to your exercise plan exactly. Second, you can always turn to other options, as long as you keep them in your training zone." She laughed, then continued philosophically, "I tend to fall into regular routines, anyway. Maybe the storm was nature's way of telling me to put a little variety in my schedule."

Week 4

During his fourth week, Brad made a bold, life-changing, move: He took a walk on the beach on Saturday. "I'm not sure what inspired me to do it—I never even look at the beach when I drive past—but somehow it just seemed like a good idea, and it was!" Assuming he continues to take weekend strolls in the future, Saturday's walk brings Brad's total weekly time-in-zone to fifty minutes of Healthy Heart time and sixty minutes of Temperate time. He got here gradually over the course of a month, and (aside from his excess enthusiasm on the stationary bike the first week) with no fatigue, discomfort, or pain for his efforts. Brad was so proud of his Week 4 plan that he posted it on his bulletin board. It looked like this:

BRAD WEEK 4	SUNDAY	MONDAY	TUESDAY	WEDNESDAY	THURSDAY	FRIDAY	SATURDAY	WEEKLY SUMMARY
ACTIVITY	Rest	Treadmill	Stair Step	Rest	Treadmill	Circuit Train	Walk	4 activities
FREQUENCY		1	1		1	1	1	5 workouts
INTENSITY		Temperate	Temperate		Temperate	Healthy Heart	Healthy Heart	2 zones
TIME		20 minutes	20 minutes		20 minutes	20 minutes	30 minutes	110 minutes

What about Brad's original goals? Well, he went in to his doctor at the end of Week 4 to get his percentage of body fat measured. Although he hesitates to reveal what his fat percentages were at the beginning or what they are now, he admits to a full 2 percent decline over the month! Brad didn't think that was a very big deal, but his doctor assured him that 2 percent represented significant progress and that, if he kept this up, he could reach a healthy percentage of body fat by the end of a year. His doctor also confirmed Brad's weight loss of six pounds and a lowering of his blood pressure, accomplishments that convinced Brad to celebrate with a new pair of workout shoes.

Brad was also realizing his other goals: logging his workouts daily and walking a mile in twenty minutes by the end of two months. According to the treadmill workout, he was now walking a comfortable mile in his Temperate zone in twenty-four minutes, a time he believed he could improve over the next month.

Marcia decided to mix things up a little with Week 4. With the weather cooperating again, she resumed her Sunday bike ride, but she decided to make her one day at the gym a regular routine as well. She also decided to stick around for the whole low-impact class this time, including the floor exercises, which kept her in the Healthy Heart zone for an extra half hour a week. This brings Marcia's weekly total time-in-zone to sixty-five minutes of Healthy Heart time and sixty minutes of Temperate zone time. She has discovered she likes to vary not only her activities but her intensities. As she told me, "With so much variety, it doesn't feel like work at all." Her Week 4 schedule looks like this:

MARCIA WEEK 4	SUNDAY	MONDAY	TUESDAY	WEDNESDAY	THURSDAY	FRIDAY	SATURDAY	WEEKLY SUMMARY
ACTIVITY	Bike	Jog	Rest	Aerobics & Floor Exercises	Rest	Jog	Rest	4 activities
FREQUENCY	1	1		1		1		4 workouts
INTENSITY	Healthy Heart	Temperate		Temperate (20 minutes) Healthy Heart (30 minutes)		Temperate		2 zones
TIME	35 minutes	20 minutes		50 minutes		20 minutes		125 minutes

How did Marcia do on her goals? Well, except for those two rainy days, she kept to her exercise schedule, working around the limitations of climate. She hasn't lost any more weight, but she definitely hasn't gained any over the course of the month, and she does find that she has slimmed down her waist and hips—the tape measure says she's lost an inch on each! Marcia said that by the end of the month, even though she had taped her goals to two bathroom mirrors she'd nearly forgotten about them; she'd gotten so caught up in how good she felt. She joked, "Maybe I'll have to change my goals for next month to something like: 'One, remember to look at your goals!'"

Continuing Weight Management

After a month of Temperate zone training, you can choose among at least two ways to go. One is to maintain your fourth week's Weight Management plan indefinitely. As long as the plan, the frequency, the intensities, and the times are getting you the results you want, there's no reason to adjust the routine. This sounds wise for Brad, who really can't afford much more time, unless he undertakes a major lifestyle change. With his Week 4 plan he can accomplish his goals quite easily.

Alternatively, you may want to make certain adjustments. Marcia may find that although she enjoys jogging and the low-impact aerobics class now, they may soon cease to challenge her. She may begin moving up the fitness curve by adding time-in-zone and spending a higher proportion of her total time-in-zone at higher intensities. If you would like to continue on a weight management program for a year, the following chart outlines a schedule you can adapt to your needs and lifestyle. This sort of program will gradually but continuously increase your FIT.

MONTH	WEEKLY TIME-IN-ZONE					
	ZONE 1 HEALTHY HEART (MINUTES)	ZONE 2 TEMPERATE (MINUTES)	ZONE 3 AEROBIC (MINUTES)	ZONE 4 THRESHOLD (MINUTES)	ZONE 5 REDLINE (MINUTES)	TOTAL WORKOUT TIME (MINUTES)
1	30	30	0	x	x	60
2	55	65	0	x	x	120
3	40	120	20	x	x	180
4	30	140	30	x	x	200
5	20	160	50	x	x	230
6	15	175	80	x	x	270
7	0	190	90	x	x	280
8	0	185	105	x	x	290
9	0	180	120	x	x	300
10	0	175	140	x	x	315
11	0	165	165	x	x	330
12	0	180	180	x	x	360

Notice that this chart allows for progress in two important categories. Month by month, total workout time per week and the number of minutes per week spent in the higher zone gradually increase. Over the course of the year workouts move out of the Healthy Heart zone and into the Aerobic zone, where all-around fitness improves as the body sheds unwanted fat and adds needed lean mass it can move more vigorously. Three factors make all the difference: Easy does it, easy does it, easy does it.

The Other Side of Weight Management: Diet

If, like Brad and Marcia, you want to win the fight against fat, then you too must follow a simple two-step program—"hanging out" in the Temperate zone, and reducing your dietary fat intake. That's all there is to it, really.

The weight-loss plan that research and experience have shown to be the most effective, commonsense, and long-term can be summarized in a single sentence:

STOP PUTTING FAT INTO YOUR BODY
BY GETTING THE FAT OUT OF YOUR DIET,
AND
GET THE FAT THAT'S ALREADY IN YOUR BODY OUT OF IT
BY TRAINING IN THE TEMPERATE ZONE.

That sentence is worth posting on your refrigerator and reading every day.

If you want to lose weight during the course of a year, you should set yourself two sensible, simple goals: reducing your fat intake to 20 to 30 percent of your total caloric intake, and reducing your body fat by exercising three or four times a week for thirty minutes a week at 60 to 70 percent Max HR.

That doesn't sound difficult, does it? It's not. If you stick with these goals, you *will* lose weight, provided you observe one caveat: Take your time. If you expect an overnight solution to your weight problem, you will be setting yourself up for yet another weight-loss disappointment. If, on the other hand, you believe that it will take as long to get the fat out as it took to get the fat in, then you will succeed, I guarantee it. In fact, for most people who put on their extra pounds gradually, over the course of years or even decades, relief will come sooner rather than later. Practicing Heart Zone Training along with smart eating can win a healthier body and a slimmer waistline for anyone.

Permanent weight loss depends on learning how to eat, not on learning how to diet. In learning to eat wisely, we deliberately select low-fat foods that provide high nutritional value. First we need to pick up some necessary skills; then we can work on changing our eating habits. Here's the bottom line, though: Eat with your brains, not your mouth and your emotions.

Weight loss experts Ronda Gates and Covert Bailey say in their book *Eat Smart* that winners in the fight against fat use intelligence when they eat. Learn what's in your food while you're learning about Heart Zone Training. You should know just as much about what you get out of the different foods you eat as you do about what you get out of the different zones in which you choose to work out.

To start, you need to count fat grams, not calories. To do this, you must read labels, keeping track of the number

of fat grams that you eat until you reach your allocation—
your "fat gram budget." Eat as much protein and carbohydrates as you want and as many fat-free calories as you like,
but—and this is a really, really big "but"—strictly limit your
intake to a fixed number of fat grams per day, based on
your total calories. If you want to eat 2,000 calories per day,
and if 25 percent of those calories come from fat, then you
need to figure out your fat budget. Since each gram of fat
contains nine calories, you calculate your budget this way:

1. Number of calories per day multiplied by 25 percent
    from fat = fat calories budget per day.
2. Fat calories per day divided by 9 calories per fat gram =
    fat gram budget per day.

For example, if you eat 2,000 calories per day, you calculate your personal budget this way:

1. 2,000 calories per day multiplied by 25 percent from fat
    = 500 fat calories per day
2. 500 fat calories per day divided by nine calories per fat
    gram = fifty-six fat grams per day.

Use the chart below to find out how many grams of fat
you can eat per day, depending on your overall caloric
intake. Remember, eat nutrient-dense foods, and when you
reach your budgeted number of grams of fat for the day, NO
MORE FAT!

THE FAT INTAKE BUDGET

CALORIES PER DAY	20% FAT (GRAMS)	30% FAT (GRAMS)
1,200	27	40
1,300	29	43
1,400	31	47
1,500	33	50
1,600	36	53
1,700	38	57
1,800	40	60
1,900	42	63
2,000	44	67
2,100	47	70
2,200	49	73
2,300	51	77
2,400	53	80
2,500	56	83
2,600	58	87
2,700	60	90
2,800	62	93
2,900	64	97
3,000	67	100

The chart begins at 1,200 calories per day, because no one can really remain healthy at fewer calories than that. (That goes for women; if you're a man, your minimum should be 1,500 calories per day.) If you're reading this book, you obviously plan to exercise, and I'll guarantee you that you're not going to be exercising without sufficient food. Circle the number of calories per day you want to set as a goal, then note your daily fat grams budget. (You may wish to get your doctor's advice about how many calories you need to be healthy.) If you plan to eat 1,700 calories daily, then your daily fat budget is thirty-eight to fifty-seven grams total. Lowering your budget any further will gain you no particular advantage, either in overall health or athletic performance. Since fat is an essential part of our diet, your health and performance depends on eating a minimum amount of it.

Remember, though, you must start writing it down. Record the number of grams of fat you eat each and every time you eat. You can keep this record in your daily planner or in your exercise log, but do keep track. Remember one of the basic Heart Zone Training principles: You can only manage what you can measure and monitor. Eating with your mind allows you to manage your weight through mental monitoring. If you want to win your own personal fat battle, you've got to pick up this crucial skill. Eventually, when you've changed the way you eat, you will no longer need to record your fat grams, because low-fat eating will have become an ingrained habit.

Get used to reading labels and buying foods marked with the words "low-fat" or "no-fat." All sorts of prepared foods meet the government's low- or no-fat criteria. Make your snack choices conscious ones: fruit, air-popped pop-corn with seasonings, diet sodas, no-oil tortilla chips, low-fat pretzels, or fat-free popsicles or cookies.

When you read labels, pay special attention to the "% Daily Value" heading and choose foods that show 5 per-cent or less in the "Total Fat" category. This way, if you eat one serving of twenty different foods per day, each totaling 5 percent or less of your total fat intake, you still won't go over 100 percent of your budgeted fat calories. Noting fat percent-ages when you shop can be easier than counting fat grams.

Get into the habit of asking questions when you buy food. For example, our local bagel bakery has a notebook with a complete nutritional breakdown for each type of bagel. However, I had to ask in order to learn that my favorite cinnamon and raisin bagel contained 360 calories and one gram of fat and that my second-favorite sesame seed bagel contained 330 calories and 1.8 grams of fat.

Make it a habit to carry food with you that fits your diet plan. Pack yourself a food bag when you leave the house—those mesh grocery bags work well. Load it up with five pieces of fruit, plenty of low-fat cookies and crackers and some carrots, and you'll never feel hungry. Trouble looms when you get hungry and lack a supply of "good" food. Your trusty good food bag can head off dietary trouble before it sends you off-course.

Your Personal Weight Management Program

You'll want to maintain two separate plans during your weight management program. The first sets your goals for the year, the second captures your weekly workout schedule.

1. In the first log, record three realistic short-term goals. They should cover between one and three months. You can modify and update them as you go along:

    Goal #1: _____

    Goal #2: _____

    Goal #3: _____

    Also write down your total calories and fat gram intake budget:
    _____ Total Calories   _____ Grams of Fat

2. You can project a full year's workout schedule here, but bear in mind that as the months go by, you will make adjustments that reflect your personal progress and evolving goals.

Sally Edwards' Heart Zone Training

HEART ZONE TRAINING LOG

	SUNDAY	MONDAY	TUESDAY	WEDNESDAY	THURSDAY	FRIDAY	SATURDAY	WEEKLY SUMMARY
ACTIVITY								
FREQUENCY								
INTENSITY								
TIME								

Achieving Optimum All-Around Fitness

Welcome to Heart Zone Training 201! Having gotten a firm grasp of the basics of Heart Zone Training in the first four chapters, you are ready to graduate to the next level of fitness and to extend the thirty-day program you designed in Chapter 2. Whether you began your program in order to feel and look better, to maintain a healthy heart, or to manage your weight, you have already embarked on a long-term journey toward optimum all-around fitness. Reaching that goal means achieving that state of physical and mental well-being that enriches everything you do in your life, be it working, playing, eating, sleeping, or just enjoying a stroll along the beach with your dog.

Optimum fitness depends on expanding your personal training program to include multiple activities in multiple zones, recording the time spent in each zone, and measuring your progress with a point system. In order to gain the best benefits from exercise, you need to progress gradually, adding steadily to your workload. To help you do that, I've developed a Heart Zone Training point system. As you tailor it to your ninety-day or long-running training program, you'll be taking into account your own particular level of fitness, your special circumstances, and your individual likes and dislikes.

For people like my neighbor Christine, a cigarette smoker who suffered "chronic exercise aversion" from repeated failures at workout programs that promised success but didn't deliver results, Heart Zone Training can make all the difference in the world. After finding out about my enthusiasm for Heart Zone Training, Christine bought a heart rate monitor and asked me to help her get started. I worried a bit at first, fearing that this might be another example of Christine's tendency to try something, not like it, and quit. Now, more than a year later, she is still reaping the benefits of Heart Zone Training. She has lost as much weight as her formerly overweight dogs, and she quit smoking because it inhibited her breathing during her Aerobic zone workouts.

Christine started exercising on the base branch of the Heart Zone Training tree. (More about that next.) After walking for four weeks in the Healthy Heart zone at 50 to 60 percent of her Max HR, she moved into a more vigorous ninety-day program, and a year later entered her first triathlon. Today she feels tremendously energetic as she works out at the club three times a week with a circuit weight program to build her strength. Our dogs have become best friends, because Christine takes them out together at least once a week for a Heart Zone Training session. Let's see how she did it.

The Training Tree

Christine optimized her fitness program by using the training tree. As a kid, I loved climbing around in the big oak trees that grow in Central California. My mom, who admired my adventuresome spirit, let me have my fun; deep down, though, she probably worried herself sick that I would fall and break a leg. With the training tree, your mother never needs to worry. It's completely safe. You go up and down and out on the limbs at your own risk, speed, and comfort levels. If you let go of a branch, you simply drop to the next limb down.

The Heart Zone Training tree looks just like a Christmas tree. The bottom branches start out big and strong, and the upper ones narrow to a point. As you climb up the training tree from the sturdy bottom branches toward the thinner, shorter ones, you'll gain more and more improvement in your all-around fitness. At each branch, you'll pause to get your balance and gather your strength before stepping up to the next level. As you climb up the training tree, spending more and more time in higher and higher zones, your body will experience wonderful changes. Think of zone climbing as your new sport!

The training tree looks like this:

THE TRAINING TREE

RACE

Choose this branch if you are training for competition.

PEAK

Choose this branch if you are preparing to race.

INTERVAL

Choose this branch if you are training to increase your speed.

STRENGTH

Choose this branch if you are training to be stronger.

ENDURANCE

Choose this branch if you are training your cardiovascular capacity.

BASE

Choose this branch if you are just starting to exercise.

RECOVERY

Choose the trunk if you are recuperating from an injury or you have overtrained.

Ready? Let's climb!

Base Branch

The first of the training tree's six branches starts with a heart-lung or cardiovascular foundation called the **base**. You have already been working out there during your initial thirty-day Heart Zone Training program. During this phase of exercise you become comfortable with the workouts, they start to feel easier, your resting and ambient heart rates drop, and you begin to see those first changes in your body as your muscles get stronger. You will want to heart zone train on the base branch for at least four to six weeks. Then, when your exercise routine begins to feel a bit too easy and you want more of a challenge, you can reach up and grab onto that next limb.

Since the base limb provides a starting point, training there should be slow, easy, and in the lowest three zones (Healthy Heart, Temperate, and Aerobic). The purpose of spending time on this branch is to develop a base level of strength and cardiovascular endurance that can sustain your workout without a great deal of fatigue and muscle soreness. It shouldn't tax you unduly or pressure you to perform beyond your capacity. Consider Christine's base program:

CHRISTINE'S THIRTY-DAY BASE PROGRAM

Activities:	Walk, bike, walk
Frequency:	3 workouts per week
Intensity (per workout):	Healthy Heart zone (10 minutes)
	Temperate zone (10 minutes)
	Aerobic zone (10 minutes)
Time:	30 minutes per workout

Notice that Christine took it slow and easy at first, engaging in activities she already enjoyed, such as walking with her dog. By the end of a month working out at the base level, she was already enjoying tangible benefits: increased calories burned per workout, increased strength, increased confidence and self esteem, improved blood pressure, easier breathing, and higher energy. Now she could comfortably climb up to the next branch.

Endurance Branch

Having base trained for a comfortable period of time, you are now ready to move up to the **endurance** limb of the tree. During this phase you will simply lengthen your time-in-zone. The endurance level is that long, slow, easy period when you move through many weeks of multiple-zone workouts and gain multiple-zone benefits. You will want to stay in the endurance phase for four to six weeks, adjusting to this new level and the longer times you spend in-zone. You will feel your body adapt to its new workload. As your muscles tone, you will find yourself able to go the same distance at a lower heart rate, while your weight stabilizes or even drops by a few pounds.

This second branch of the tree develops your cardiovascular system's ability to sustain longer periods of training. Technically speaking, your body can now carry more oxygen to your muscles and break into your fat storage cells to burn calories. Not only does your heart beat more strongly, each beat expels more blood, and your blood vessels open more widely. Here's how Christine did it:

CHRISTINE'S NINETY-DAY ENDURANCE PROGRAM	
Activities:	Walk, run, bike, walk, low-impact aerobics
Frequency:	5 workouts per week
Intensity (per workout):	Healthy Heart zone (5 minutes)
	Temperate zone (10 minutes)
	Aerobic zone (15 minutes)
Time:	30 minutes per workout

Ready for more of a challenge, Christine adds a couple more strenuous workouts to her program, a run and an aerobics class. She also spends more time now in the higher Aerobic zone. Well before the end of this three-month period she gains these benefits: More effective use of oxygen, stronger muscles capable of moving more easily for longer periods of time, and a heart pumping more blood to more vessels. Now Christine can boost herself up to the next branch on the training tree: She is heart-healthy.

Strength Branch

On the **strength** branch of the training tree you will add what fitness folks call "resistance" training. Resistance, or strength, training makes your muscles stronger and more powerful but not necessarily faster. Workouts on the strength limb include activities like walking up hills, running, climbing stairs, and weight training with machines or free weights. On the strength limb you can add high-tech toys like cross-training machines, isokinetic swim benches, or cycling wind trainers—or you can perform simple calisthenics like push-ups, dips, and sit-ups.

The purpose of the strength phase is to build strength in specific muscles. If you like to swim, you might add training devices such as fins and hand paddles or swim buoys, which you place between your thighs. These training aids work your muscles harder but do not necessarily make you faster. If you're a runner or cyclist, you can add hills during your strength-training period.

By putting more weight or work on a muscle, you make it stronger. As muscles get stronger, they can generate a greater force. Resistance training such as weight lifting applies an "overload principle" to exercise. When you load the muscle with more weight than it normally handles, it will respond by fatiguing first and then recovering to a stronger point than before the overload occurred.

Fitness experts always advise using this training technique at a slow rate and with few repetitions. For example, you might start by lifting a two-pound weight ten times until that becomes easy. Then add either repetitions (reps) or weight. You can lift two pounds twelve times (repetitions) or three pounds ten times. In either case, your muscles recognize an overload and respond accordingly.

I do one of my favorite strength workouts in a tall office building with air-conditioned stairwells. Strapping on my heart rate monitor, I walk up and down the flights of stairs, trying to stay in my Aerobic zone for twenty minutes. It's hard to maintain this heart rate because I always want to race up and walk slowly down, but I love the feeling I get when my legs are feeling the burn, because I know the next day they will be stronger from my strength workouts. Here's what Christine did:

CHRISTINE'S SIXTY-DAY STRENGTH PROGRAM

Activities:	Walk/run, run, bike, walk/run, Threshold zone
Frequency:	5 workouts per week
Intensity (per workout):	Healthy Heart zone (5 minutes) Temperate zone (10 minutes) Aerobic zone (20 minutes) Threshold zone (5 minutes)
Time:	40 minutes per workout

Not only did Christine lengthen her workout sessions from thirty to forty minutes, she increased her intensity to get her, for the first time and briefly, into the higher Threshold zone, and she made her walking, cycling, and aerobics more strenuous. During this phase of her training she obtained these benefits: stronger and more well-toned muscles.

Before Christine—or you—consider going out on the next limb of the training tree, I must offer a word of caution. The next three branches apply to people who desire performance benefits. For most of us, optimum all-around fitness does not require training ourselves into high-performance athletes. If you do set that goal for yourself, then you will not only climb the next three branches, you will want to study Chapter 7, "Reaching the Most Advanced Level of Heart Zone Training," where I offer advice for the genuine competitor. Since Christine decided to stay on the lower branches of the training tree, I will not apply them to her program.

Interval Branch

On the **interval** limb you design a program that will enable you to get faster, which is a great feeling. You'll begin your first "interval" training sessions, measuring elapsed time, distance, and heart rate together. During this speed phase you will learn about "pick-ups," or surges, and what Swedish trainers call "fartleks," or "speed play." See the creative speed workouts in Chapter 6 and pick ones for your favorite sports. Remember that Heart Zone Training is universal—it works for all sports, all activities, and all people.

As your body reaps benefits from your work on the interval branch, you'll be able to go faster and cover longer distances in less time while your heart rate stays the same. It's a wonderful feeling to become more fleet-footed with less stress and strain. You'll almost feel the walls of your vessels open up and the blood surge through them.

This phase of training builds upon the lower three branches by adding Redline zone workouts with short and long sprints or intervals. It produces high heart rate numbers as you are pushed ever closer to your Max HR. It's a time when you breathe hard, stare at the face of the monitor, and watch the heart rate numbers climb to the upper limits of the top zone. You'll "feel the burn" from going really hard and really fast, but in return you get faster.

There's a saying among athletes: "If you want to get fast, train fast. If you want to train fast, redline." Whenever you redline, you move into a danger zone, and so it's crucial to limit the amount of time spent in that zone. That's interval training—mixing fast and hard with slow and easy in one workout. You get faster.

Peak Branch

The fifth branch earns the label **peak** because it's here that you reach your highest level of fitness, preparing yourself for your own peak performance. It's a key branch for high-level athletic performance. It's a narrow and short limb, however you can't stay on it forever, because it's not as strong as the branches below. The training tree requires you to move up—and down—by providing opportunities for different training times and intensities on each branch. That variety, the spice of life in exercise, provides the body with the changes it needs to improve.

The peak branch, and the one above it, exist only for those who want to test their mettle against others, to expand themselves in the world of "How fast can I go?" or "How long can I endure?" Don't worry about this branch unless you consider yourself a serious athlete and want to race at your best.

Race Branch

The **race** branch marks the top of the tree. Reach for it only if you want to find out what it feels like to be maximally fit; this one applies to competitors who want top performance benefits from their training program. Those who reach this branch want to experience their own peak performance, try for a faster time, finish stronger, or earn a personal record. Climbing up onto the racing branch makes no sense for those who seek health and fitness benefits like losing weight or getting fit. In other words, there is a difference between an athlete and a competitor. Anyone who works out is an athlete. If you heart zone train, you are an athlete. If you exercise regularly, you are an athlete. Anyone can become an athlete. Competitors, on the other hand, want to challenge themselves to the utmost. They race against a finish line clock, against others in the race. Athletes race against themselves and their personal performance.

Recovery Trunk

You may have been wondering why I saved the trunk of the tree, **recovery**, for last. It's because the recovery trunk serves a vital function for all heart zone trainers, from those who hang out on the lowest branch to those who reach the very top. It is especially essential, however, for anyone who climbs up to the higher branches, where the oxygen grows thin and the height of the tree can become exhausting.

With this tree, of course, you need not climb down through the lower limbs to reach the trunk. Just shimmy on down, hang out, and rest. The recovery trunk allows the body to exercise and rest simultaneously. Recovery is a training phase or period. By staying in very low heart zones for short "recovery" workouts, you recuperate from the climb, especially the long climb to the top of the tree. You may get a little unfit during this resting period, but every body needs some recovery before starting back up the training tree.

Don't think for a moment that you can swing in the top of the tree forever. The body has its limits. Many of you probably know someone like Ron at my gym. We call him "the animal." His training schedules border on the obsessive, and he can race with the best of them. He spends hours in his upper heart zones and races hard week after week. Ron will *never* leave the top of the tree by choice, but his frequent injuries from overtraining and incessant racing put him on the ground nonetheless. I prefer to plan my recoveries and build them into my training tree schedule. All heart zoners, from those on the lower branches to serious competitors, should do the same.

Let's put it all together now. The tree on the next page shows the amount of time you should plan to spend in each zone for the branch you have selected for yourself:

Time-In-Zone as a Percentage

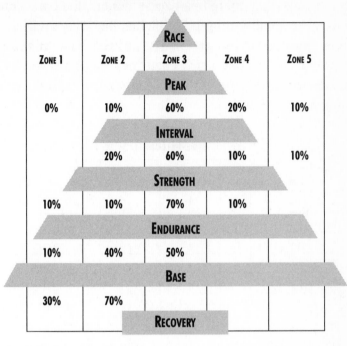

Zone 1	Zone 2	Zone 3	Zone 4	Zone 5
		RACE		
0%	10%	PEAK 60%	20%	10%
	20%	INTERVAL 60%	10%	10%
10%	10%	STRENGTH 70%	10%	
10%	40%	ENDURANCE 50%		
30%	70%	BASE		
		RECOVERY		

With these bases in mind, let's do it!

Beginning the Climb

Having learned the basic training tree concepts, you can now put yourself on one of the limbs and begin your climb. Those of you who are already training may find yourself starting on one of the middle branches. That's fine. You only have to start at the recovery trunk if you are totally new to exercise or just recovering from an injury or all-important race. For most beginning heart zone trainers, the base branch provides the ideal starting point. Remember, safe and healthy exercise must progress gradually, and the base guarantees that. The Time-In-Zone (TIZ) chart indicates how you might allocate your training time to each zone based on the training tree branch:

TIME-IN-ZONE

ZONE	MAX HR	TRAINING ZONE	TIME IN BASE ZONE		TIME IN ENDURANCE ZONE		TIME IN STRENGTH ZONE		TIME IN INTERVAL ZONE		TIME IN PEAK/RACE ZONE	
Z5	90–100%	Redline	—		—		—		10%		10%	
Z4	80–90%	Threshold	—		—		10%		10%		20%	
Z3	70–80%	Aerobic	—		50%		70%		60%		60%	
Z2	60–70%	Temperate	70%		40%		10%		20%		10%	
Z1	50–60%	Healthy Heart	30%		10%		10%				—	
				Min.	100%	Min.	100%	Min.	100%	Min.	100%	Min.

Lets say you plan to begin a single-sport exercise program such as cycling. Before getting on a bike, be sure it's in good working condition, and check the tires and brakes. If you aren't in great shape, or if you have not cycled recently, start on the base limb, spending all of your riding time for at least the first two weeks in the lowest zones. Ride for ten to twenty minutes in the Healthy Heart and Temperate zones. Use these beginning workouts to become comfortable with your bike-handling skills. As you grow more proficient, riding longer and at higher heart rates will automatically become easier and more enjoyable. Here's how a four-week base cycling program might look:

SAMPLE TRAINING PROGRAM: BASE BRANCH

WEEK NUMBER	ACTIVITY	ZONES	TIME-IN-ZONE (TIZ)
#1	Bike	Healthy Heart Temperate	10–20 minutes 15–25 minutes
#2	Bike	Healthy Heart Temperate	10–20 minutes 20–25 minutes
#3 and #4	Bike	Healthy Heart Temperate	10–25 minutes 35–55 minutes

Feel free to experiment. Your own training tree belongs only to you—it's yours to nourish, grow, or trim to match your goals. Fitness programs today, unlike in the past, take the individual into account. What works for you only works for you. As you plan your ascent up the tree, don't just follow the written programs outlined in this book. Personalize your plan to match your schedule, your work week, your lifestyle, and your goals.

You'll appreciate the training tree more fully when I explain how to use your time-in-zone to maintain a Heart Zone Training personal log. Then all the pieces will come together. For now, let's stay on the base branch. If you're a beginner, the base branch is a challenging and fun place to work out. You will begin to see the benefits of exercise translated into your body as you walk up the stairs more easily, feel more energy, sleep better, and boost your self-esteem. But the base limb is not just for beginners! Last summer an Arabian horse and I got into a tangle over who was in charge, and we both went down. Unfortunately, the wrong one of us ended up on the bottom. When the horse reared and rolled backward, trying to throw me, I recognized this smart aleck equine trick and threw myself out of the way, but not far enough. The horse landed on my Achilles tendon, tearing it severely and putting me out of training for months. Returning to training, I vowed not to reinjure myself. I trained at 50 to 70 percent of Max HR for four weeks and gradually, ever so gradually, built back both my Achilles tendon and my heart. By staying comfortable and slow, I was able to return to my racing form and progressively climb back up my training tree. I love that tree. I love climbing it most of all. I love reaching the top.

The Heart Zone Training Point System

Would you like to keep track of all of your heart zone exercise in a handy way? Would you like an integrated "system" that fits your individual situation? I've developed just such a device; I call it the Heart Zone Training Point System. Recall my earlier observation that you can only manage what you can measure and monitor. That's what the system provides, a simple tool to measure and monitor your workouts, tracking and logging them so that you will know exactly how much time you spend in each of the five training zones. It's also a reward mechanism, awarding more points as you gradually spend more time in a zone or exercise in higher zones.

The Heart Zone Training Point System employs a simple daily log. As you record your daily activity and award yourself points, you become motivated to hit your weekly and monthly goals. Accumulating points can drive your Heart Zone Training program. In addition to giving you a way to manage your program, the system also quantifies your workload precisely and provides an accurate assessment tool for understanding it. You want to focus on workload, because it sums up the FIT formula discussed in Chapter 1.

The Heart Zone Training Point System works like this:

- You earn one point for every one minute of exercise.
- You earn additional points by working out in the various zones.

ZONE	POINTS	ZONE NUMBER
Redline	5	Z5
Threshold	4	Z4
Aerobic	3	Z3
Temperate	2	Z2
Healthy Heart	1	Z1

- You multiply your points by the zone number for a daily total.
- You add your daily totals to calculate weekly point totals.

Last week I earned 180 points by engaging in three thirty-minute workouts in three different zones:

Sally Edwards' Heart Zone Training

HEART ZONE TRAINING POINTS LOG

	MONTH/DATE	SPORT ACTIVITY	Z1	Z2	Z3	Z4	Z5	TOTAL POINTS	DAILY NOTES	COMMENTS
					TIME IN ZONES					
MONDAY	3/3	Walk	30					30	Resting HR: 68 / Weight: 139 / Other:	Windy & cold / Easy pace
TUESDAY	3/4								Resting HR: / Weight: / Other:	
WEDNESDAY	3/5	Bike		30				60	Resting HR: 70 / Weight: 141 / Other:	Indoors / 130 bpm
THURSDAY	3/6								Resting HR: / Weight: / Other:	
FRIDAY	3/7	Swim			30			90	Resting HR: 67 / Weight: 140 / Other:	Water warm / Coach missed practice
SATURDAY	3/8								Resting HR: / Weight: / Other:	
SUNDAY	3/9								Resting HR: / Weight: / Other:	
			30	30	30			180	WEEKLY HZT POINTS TOTAL	
			Z1	Z2	Z3	Z4	Z5			

ZONE NAME	ZONE POINTS	% OF MAX HR
Redline Zone	5	100–90%
Threshold Zone	4	90–80%
Aerobic Zone	3	80–70%
Temperate Zone	2	70–60%
Healthy Heart Zone	1	60–50%

Total Weekly HZT Points: Multiply the time in each zone by the number of that zone.

Achieving Optimum All-Around Fitness

HEART ZONE TRAINING POINTS LOG

MONTH/ DATE	SPORT ACTIVITY	TIME IN ZONES					TOTAL POINTS	DAILY NOTES	COMMENTS
		Z1	Z2	Z3	Z4	Z5			
MONDAY								Resting HR: Weight: Other:	
TUESDAY								Resting HR: Weight: Other:	
WEDNESDAY								Resting HR: Weight: Other:	
THURSDAY								Resting HR: Weight: Other:	
FRIDAY								Resting HR: Weight: Other:	
SATURDAY								Resting HR: Weight: Other:	
SUNDAY								Resting HR: Weight: Other:	
								WEEKLY HZT POINTS TOTAL	
		Z1	Z2	Z3	Z4	Z5			
								% TIZ	

Total Weekly HZT Points: Multiply the time in each zone by the number of that zone.

ZONE NAME	ZONE POINTS	% OF MAX HR
Redline Zone	5	100–90%
Threshold Zone	4	90–80%
Aerobic Zone	3	80–70%
Temperate Zone	2	70–60%
Healthy Heart Zone	1	60–50%

The Heart Zone Training Point System applies to all workouts in all sports and zones. For example, five minutes of cycling in the Aerobic zone (Z3) equals five minutes of swimming in the same zone. As far as the workout's value goes, it doesn't matter whether you are hiking, snow boarding, scuba diving, or playing squash. What's important is the amount of time you spend in-zone and the numerical values of that zone. I'll explore this point further in the next chapter, but at this point merely bear in mind that as you exercise in each of the five different zones, you earn different benefits and different point scores depending on your heart rate intensity and the amount of time you spend in-zone. All you have to do is set your training zones and times-in-zone at the beginning of the workout, then stay within those zones for the set amount of time.

Within a year of starting her Heart Zone Training program, my neighbor Christine had worked up to 250 points a week, when back surgery curtailed her workouts. Proud of her progress and the fact that she had finally kicked the nicotine habit, Christine hated this unexpected setback. Ironically, her operation provided an interesting learning experience. When Christine received medical clearance to exercise, she started by walking sixty minutes a day in the Healthy Heart zone (Z1), earning sixty points per day. Within two weeks Christine progressed to walking three hours(180 minutes) a day in the same zone, logging 180 points per day. Unfortunately, she tried doing too much too soon, overextended herself, and had to stop when her back pain reappeared. Six months later Christine needed another back operation.

The second time around she started her exercise program smarter and more conservatively. Beginning at the recovery trunk of the training tree, Christine earned 100 points a week, budgeting herself for no more than twenty-five points in any one day. After a month of recovery workout, she started climbing up the tree. Six months later Christine finished her first all-women's Danskin Triathlon race. For the first time in her life she swam half a mile, biked twelve miles, and ran/walked 3.1 miles. You couldn't keep the smile off of her face or the finisher's t-shirt off of her back for weeks.

Your total points per week and month should become both a goal and an accomplishment. Let's look at Jennifer—the engineer from Chapter 2—when she was in her second week of training. Here's her workout schedule again, with Heart Zone Training points added to it:

HEART ZONE TRAINING POINTS LOG

DAY	SPORT	ZONE	ZONE NUMBER	TIME	HZT POINTS
MONDAY	Rest				
TUESDAY	Bike	Temperate	2	20	40
WEDNESDAY	Rest				
THURSDAY	Walk	Healthy Heart	1	20	20
FRIDAY	Rest				
SATURDAY	Bike	Temperate	2	20	40
SUNDAY	Tennis	Healthy Heart	1	40	40
				Total:	140 points

To complete the Heart Zone Training Points Log at the end of this chapter, you must decide how many points you want to earn for the week. What point goal should you set? That depends on several factors. Are you already training, or have you recently begun a program? What goals do you want to shoot for? What would you like to accomplish? When do you want to accomplish your first goal? If you have already launched an exercise or training program, just log your current workouts and calculate how many points you average on a weekly basis. This will give you some basic facts to get you started. If you've been keeping a record of your workouts, go back and review the last several months and add your points per week.

If this is your first day of Heart Zone Training, begin easy and progress gradually by setting a goal of 100 points a week. Divide your 100 points between the number of days on which you will engage in cardiovascular workouts. If you plan to train four days a week, you'll aim for twenty-five points per day on the average, or twenty-five minutes in Z1 (Healthy Heart zone) for four days. If you want to do both Z1 and Z2 sessions, then calculate the points accordingly. The previous example totaled 160 points per week, perhaps a little high for some beginners.

Next, decide where you sit on the training tree. If you are already training and have set goals, you may have progressed above the base branch. If you are brand-new to exercise, then plan to spend 100 percent of your time in the Healthy Heart zone on the base branch. As you climb up the training tree, you will be spending more time-in-zone, earning more and more points and getting fitter and fitter all the time.

An advanced Heart Zone Trainer may earn 1,000 points a week or even more. I know a number of Olympic-caliber athletes who train as much as 6,000 points a week, far beyond the needs of most everyone except those pursuing elite, gold-medal competitive goals.

The following suggested totals, based on athletic background and experience, may help you set your training point goals:

FITNESS LEVEL	WEEKLY HEART ZONE TRAINING POINTS
Not in shape	75–100 points
Exercising 1 or 2 days or under 2 hours/week	75–150 points
Working out 3 days or under 3 hours/week	100–200 points
Exercising daily	150–400 points
Training regularly	200–500 points
Training for a race	300–750 points
Training for a longer race	500–1,000 points
Elite or high-level competition	1,000-plus points

Sally's 1,000-Point Weekly HZT Program

To give you an idea of how I develop a multi-sport, multi-zone training plan, I'd like to share with you my own 1,000-point workout week. On Monday I like to ride my mountain bike for an hour in my Temperate zone. Since I'm exercising in Z2, I multiply the 60 minutes by 2 and earn 120 points. This is a steady-state heart rate (SSHR) workout for me, so I try to stay at or around the middle of that zone. **Points: 120**.

Tuesday is my interval day, where I train in two different zones. I usually run long intervals for one-mile segments with a large Sacramento running club called the Buffalo Chips. Since the club includes different pace groups, I choose the one that fits my heart rate, not my leg speed. I usually join the group that runs a 6:15 to 6:30-minute mile for each of the four miles and walk/jogs a quarter-mile for an active rest between miles. My recovery heart rate during the rest drops as low as 120 bpm, the middle of my Temperate zone. I usually set my planned workout zone to 180 to 185 bpm for a Redline interval session. Points for Tuesday include forty points for eight minutes of warm-up and twelve minutes of active rest in Z2 and twenty-six minutes in Z5. **Total Points: 170**.

Wednesday I swim. I like to warm up for 200 yards and then swim three sets of 500 yards (usually I mix strokes, but sometimes I do all freestyle) at a steady-state heart rate (SSHR) intensity in the middle of my Aerobic zone, Z3. It's a comfortable swim, and I feel great for the whole forty-minute workout. **Total points: 120**.

I go on a group bike ride most Thursday afternoons. Three of us leave from downtown and take off for a twenty-five-mile ride in the country. It takes a long thirty-minute warm-up to get out of the city; then we have some fun doing pace-line training on country roads. We enjoy a long cool-down as we cruise back through town. Average heart rate is not a good indicator for this workout, because the ride to the outskirts of town with stoplights and cars falls in Z1, the Healthy Heart zone, while the pace-line work falls in Z4, the Threshold zone, for about thirty minutes. **Total Points: 180**.

Friday is a rest day or a day when I do some alternative kind of exercise, such as extra stretching or extra weight training.

Saturday I usually devote to a race or a fun run, and I choose a zone based on what training stage I'm in at the time. In this case I picked an SSHR easy aerobic run in Z3 that took about fifty minutes. **Total Points: 150**.

On Sunday I like to do a double workout. I might do back-to-back training sessions such as bike-runs, biking for one hour and then running for one hour in Z3. Since my Max HR on the bike is ten beats lower than when I run, I must adjust the zones on my monitor. **Total Points: 360.**

This is my typical training schedule at the middle of my training progression, when I'm on the interval branch of the training tree. My total training time for the week is 6.5 hours, or just under an hour a day, which I can easily fit into my work schedule. I also find that this program allows me to race well and remain injury-free. Here's how I filled out my planning log:

Sally Edwards' Heart Zone Training

HEART ZONE TRAINING POINTS LOG

	MONTH/DATE	SPORT ACTIVITY	Z1	Z2	Z3	Z4	Z5	TOTAL POINTS
					TIME IN ZONES			
MONDAY	2/12	Mountain Bike		60				120
TUESDAY	2/13	Run Interval		20			26	170
WEDNESDAY	2/14	Swim			40			120
THURSDAY	2/15	Bike	60			30		180
FRIDAY	2/16	Rest!						
SATURDAY	2/17	Run			50			150
SUNDAY	2/18	Bike Run			60 60			360
			60	80	210	30	26	1100
			Z1	Z2	Z3	Z4	Z5	WEEKLY HZT POINTS TOTAL
			15%	20%	50%	8%	8%	100% % TIZ

ZONE NAME	ZONE POINTS	% OF MAX HR
Redline Zone	5	100–90%
Threshold Zone	4	90–80%
Aerobic Zone	3	80–70%
Temperate Zone	2	70–60%
Healthy Heart Zone	1	60–50%

Total Weekly HZT Points: Multiply the time in each zone by the number of that zone.

Your Personal Log

Now it's time to think about goals, pick your branch of the training tree, and complete the first page of your Heart Zone Training planner log. You may want to refer to the training tree diagram on page 102 and the TIZ chart on page 111.

Date: _____

My climb up the training tree will start at the _____ branch.

My time-in-zone(s) for this branch include:

Zone Name(s)	Percent of Time
_____	_____
_____	_____
_____	_____
_____	_____
_____	_____

I can devote _____ minutes per week to my Heart Zone Training program.

My goal is to earn _____ Heart Zone Training points per week by doing _____ workouts as shown in the planner log on the next page.

Sally Edwards' Heart Zone Training

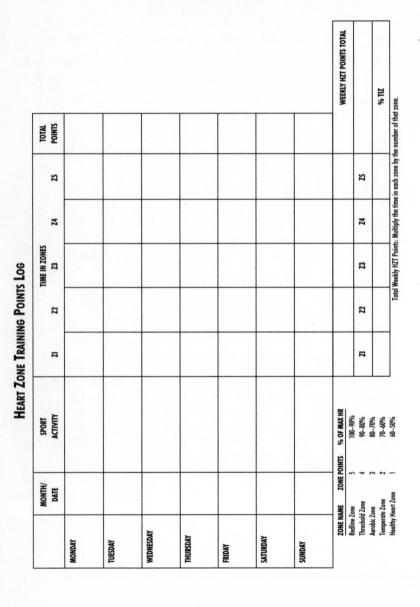

HEART ZONE TRAINING POINTS LOG

| MONTH/ DATE | SPORT ACTIVITY | TIME IN ZONES | | | | | TOTAL POINTS | WEEKLY HZT POINTS TOTAL |
		Z1	Z2	Z3	Z4	Z5		
MONDAY								
TUESDAY								
WEDNESDAY								
THURSDAY								
FRIDAY								
SATURDAY								
SUNDAY								
		Z1	Z2	Z3	Z4	Z5		
								% TIZ

ZONE NAME	ZONE POINTS	% OF MAX HR
Redline Zone	5	100–90%
Threshold Zone	4	90–80%
Aerobic Zone	3	80–70%
Temperate Zone	2	70–60%
Healthy Heart Zone	1	60–50%

Total Weekly HZT Points: Multiply the time in each zone by the number of that zone.

You know what they say about the "best-laid plans of mice and (wo)men." Since lack of time can always get in the way of our plans, I suggest you get a log plan, then record what you actually accomplish. You can always make adjustments to your plan when lifestyle or work changes come into your life, without giving up your goal of achieving optimum all-around fitness.

Getting Creative with Your Fitness Program

My friend Michael can always make me laugh. He's a freelance writer who lives in rural Massachusetts, and since he had recently began working out with a heart rate monitor, I called him up to ask for his help. "Hey, Michael, you're a creative guy; help me out here. I'm writing a chapter on getting creative with a fitness program, and I need some fun, non-sports stuff."

A week later he called me back, saying he'd worn his monitor from the minute he got out of bed one day until he went to sleep that night. "It was pretty amazing," he said. "Some activities boosted my heart rate more than I figured they would, others did it less."

He went on to say that when he went outside to shovel four inches of new-fallen snow off his driveway, his heart rate shot up to 142 in less than ten minutes, well into his Z4

Threshold zone. "No wonder doctors tell people to take it easy with the snow shovel," Michael marveled.

An indoor doubles tennis match late that morning hardly raised his heart rate at all. "Free-serving and rushing the net, I never got my rate over 110, the middle of my Z1 Temperate zone. So I got on that rowing machine at the club, and, wow, I got into my Z3 Aerobic zone in no time flat. I'm going to hit the club twenty minutes early from now on and pump those oars before I play tennis."

Splitting firewood got Michael into his Aerobic zone, too, but romping with his dog in the snow kept him down in the Z2 Temperate. "OK," I said, "tell me something I don't know."

He laughed. "Two things, Sal. My wife and I took a little nap in the afternoon, and one thing led to another and, boom, 110, Z1 Healthy Heart zone. I'm definitely adding sex to my exercise program. But *this* really amazed me: When I came in after shoveling the driveway, I was breathing hard and sweating, and wouldn't you know it, the phone rang and I had to talk to the editor who'd called. When I took three deep breaths, looking at my monitor, I saw my heart rate drop almost magically from 110 to 95. What about using your monitor for relaxation, meditation, and stress reduction?"

Do what Michael did. Wear your monitor for a full day, or, if you haven't bought one yet, take your pulse during all sorts of activities. Try something new, like those exercise machines you've gotten curious about. Have fun, get creative.

I practice what I preach. My friend and training partner, Heidi, learned about my passion for Heart Zone Training during one of our first workouts together. Her running coach had told her that in order to become a great runner she should *only* run. He taught Heidi that she needed to run "hard" one day and run "easy" the next day for a certain number of miles. She thought that hard meant running as fast as she could go and that easy meant she could just casually lope along.

At the beginning of our workout, I announced my own personal plan. "Today is an upper Z4 Threshold zone cycling workout at 175 to 180 bpm." She looked at me as if I had just spoken to her in a foreign language, then shook her head, grinned, and strapped on the heart rate monitor I'd brought along for her. When we took off on our bikes, Heidi could only sustain the pace for about 15 minutes before she suggested we slow down. That ruined my plan, but it did give us a chance to talk about training in zones, training with a written plan, training with a goal, and the great feeling you get by accomplishing your goal.

The next day I said I was running and swimming and doing a "double"—two workouts in one day. As I told her about my multiple zones, I could see that it was all starting to make sense to her. When Heidi finally put it all together, she said, "Sally, you train less time and get more benefit than I do. Right?" Right. Heidi decided to try my method. Once she started cross-training with her monitor, she actually became a faster runner.

You should do the same. By cross-training, working with a plan and using multiple zones to get multiple benefits, you can get creative with your own unique program. You'll also get fitter, you'll get faster, and you'll get a tremendous emotional charge from your training.

Creative HZT Training Programs

To keep the fun in your Heart Zone Training, you should continue to try new activities, or do the same old activities in different ways. Cross-train indoors as well as outdoors. Lift weights or try resistance training, stretch your muscles to increase their range of motion. Take up new activities that spark your curiosity, challenging yourself with the question, "When was the *last time* I did something for the *first time?*"

Here are some suggestions for putting more fun in your outdoor and indoor activities.

Zone Play

This works like *fartlek*, the Swedish term for "speed play," and it means that you do quick pick-ups or short spurts of speed and then recover by slowing down before you go fast again. During zone play you pick two single heart-rate points—a high one and a low one—and make sure you get your heart rate up and down, hitting your numbers. For instance, I sometimes pick the numbers 140 and 170. Other times I prefer to work in my Redline zone, so I'll choose 165 and 185. After picking your own numbers, determine a total training time, such as thirty minutes. Now go off and play, bouncing back and forth between the two numbers. Speed up until your heart rate reaches the high point, then slow to an easy pace until it drops to the low point. Enable the audible alarm on your heart rate monitor to sound off when you hit your numbers. Keep doing that between the two heart rate points for the entire workout time. On a treadmill you can run, then walk, then run, then walk. Or, as Michael did, shovel snow, then toss a frisbee to your dog.

Criss-Cross Conditioning

I like to do this workout in my Z3 Aerobic zone on one day and my Z4 Threshold zone on another. I'll spend five minutes at the ceiling of my Aerobic zone (155 bpm), then slow down for five minutes at the floor or bottom of my Aerobic zone (140 bpm) before speeding up and reaching the ceiling again. On an alternate day I pick my Z4 Threshold zone, 155 to 175 bpm, and bounce between those two numbers. I cycle at each number for five minutes before changing. You can do the same running, walking, climbing stairs, chopping wood, planting the garden, or dancing.

Steady-State Points

With steady-state points you select a single heart rate number, such as 145 bpm, within a given zone, such as 135 to 155 bpm. I love this kind of exercise session, because it really makes me work to hold my heart rate at that single number. I usually pick the mid-point in one of my five zones as the best number. Given my Max HR of 200 bpm, my zone midpoints look like this:

ZONE NUMBER	ZONE NAME	ZONE RANGE (MY MAX HR IS 195 BPM)	ZONE MIDPOINT
Z5	Redline	180–200	190
Z4	Threshold	160–180	170
Z3	Aerobic	140–160	150
Z2	Temperate	120–140	130
Z1	Healthy Heart	100–120	110

Take a few minutes to write your Max HR and zone ranges below, then calculate your own mid-point heart rates so you can set them as future reference points:

ZONE NUMBER	ZONE NAME	ZONE RANGE (MY MAX HR IS _____ BPM)	ZONE MIDPOINT
Z5	Redline		
Z4	Threshold		
Z3	Aerobic		
Z2	Temperate		
Z1	Healthy Heart		

When I am training for competition, I do steady-state heart rate training two days a week. One of those days I run for the entire period at Threshold zone midpoint, using the number 170 as my steady-state point. Throughout the workout I try to stay as close to that number as possible. On the other day I choose a different activity, such as cycling, and I'll try to stay in the Z2 Temperate zone, using the 130 bpm midpoint. I "spin" or cycle easily at that number for the entire workout and feel refreshed at the end. Michael picked rowing for one day's steady workout at 138 bpm, and doubles tennis for one day at 106 bpm—the midpoints of his Z4 Threshold and Z2 Temperate zones.

Flexibility Rates

I strongly recommend adding stretching exercises to your Heart Zone Training, simply because it contributes so much to your all-around fitness. When you stretch, your joints become more limber and your range of motion increases. This means that the next time you bend over to pull up a pair of socks, you'll find it much easier to reach your feet. When you want to reach behind your back to fasten on your heart rate monitor or rub a sore muscle, you'll be able to do that more easily too.

Be sure to stretch only when you have "warmed up" the muscle in question by gently and methodically exercising the specific body area to get blood actively flowing through it. If you are going to stretch your lower body, for example, ride an exercise bike for five minutes or walk for the same time to warm up. Then, keep checking your heart rate numbers as you try the following five stretching exercises, watching the numbers on your monitor as they change. Stretching is activity-specific, so the stretches that runners do are different from those golfers do. These, however, are general, all-purpose stretches for you to try using your heart rate monitor:

1. *Torso Stretch*: Sit in a straight position on the floor and straighten out your left leg. Wrap your left arm around your bent right knee and gently press the knee toward your chest. Keep your back straight and your right palm flat on the floor behind your back as you look over your right shoulder and breathe deeply. Stretch the opposite side in the same position. Look at your monitor each time.

2. *Inner Thigh Stretch*: From a standing position, start by bending your knees as you place your hands on the floor in front of you. Sliding your left leg out to the side as you bend your right knee, lower your hips with your arms inside your legs. Your right elbow presses your right knee outward; your right heel should be on the floor. Hold for ten seconds, stand, and bend your knees this time with the right leg out to the side. Look at your monitor each time.

3. *Shoulder Stretch*: Stand straight, bend your right arm behind your head, and press your right elbow downward with your left hand. Hold for five seconds and repeat with the left. Look at your monitor each time.

4. *Elongation Stretch*: Lie on your back, extend your arms overhead, and simultaneously point your toes. Stretch as far as possible, pointing your hands and toes. Hold for ten seconds and relax. Look at your monitor each time.

5. *Quadricep ("Quad") Stretch*: In a standing position, use your left hand to pull your right foot towards your buttock; hold the foot so that you're balancing on one leg. Hold the stretch for ten to twenty seconds, then repeat with the opposite leg. Look at your monitor each time.

Michael uses yoga exercises to increase his flexibility, keeping his heart rate at around 100 bpm, the lower end of his Z2 Temperate zone. Dancing, calisthenics, and any other stretching moves can achieve the same effect for you.

Fifty-Beat Interval Workouts

Fifty-beat interval workouts are another form of hard-easy exercise, but this highly-structured technique gets your heart rate moving among three zones instead of two. Identify a fifty-beat zone, such as 130 to 180, warm up, increase your activity until you hit the top number, then immediately slow down until you drop down fifty beats. Repeat this process five times. Michael found it easy to perform his fifty-beat interval on the rowing machine, but you can do it just as easily with your favorite activity, provided it allows for the full fifty-beat range. You can use other ranges as well, varying the day and the range. I use a twenty-five–beat range one day and a forty-beat interval range.

Zone Ladders

Zone Ladders is one of my favorite workouts, because it takes my heart rate through four zones, like climbing four rungs of a ladder. Start with a five-minute warm-up in Z1, the Healthy Heart zone. Next, pick up the pace ever so slightly until you get into Z2, the Temperate zone, and stay there for five minutes. At the end of that period, step up into Z3, the Aerobic zone, for five minutes. Now, either go back down the ladder in five-minute steps or take one more step up into Z4, the Threshold zone, staying there for five minutes. During that last step you might find yourself breathing hard and sweating profusely. Whenever you feel too heavily taxed, go back down the ladder. "It took me three months to do a four-rung ladder workout comfortably," says Michael. "You were right about taking it easy, but I finally did get there, and those five minutes in Z4 have given me much more stamina on the tennis court."

Progression Accents

Progression Accents is another ladder workout, but with this one you only move up the ladder, not down. It's one of the most challenging workouts because you work harder the higher you climb. With each step up you drop one minute of time:

ZONE	TIME-IN-ZONE
Z1	5 minutes
Z2	4 minutes
Z3	3 minutes
Z4	2 minutes
Z5	1 minute

Indoor Cross-Training

Most people these days engage in some sort of indoor exercising, either at home or in a club. It's easy, safe, fun, and social; it also provides a helpful structure or discipline in which to exercise. Many indoor enthusiasts have discovered that they love a certain piece of exercise equipment so much that they tend to spend all of their time on that one piece of machinery, be it a climbing machine, a recumbent bike, a rowing machine, a cross-country skiing machine, or a stationary bicycle. These are all wonderful contraptions, but most have one drawback: The manufacturers have preprogrammed them with so-called "typical" variables. That's nonsense. You're a unique individual with your own set of heart rate zones. Even though I am almost fifty years old, when I use pre-programmed equipment, I always have to input twenty-three years old when a machine asks for my age. You too may need to "override" your favorite machine to tailor it to your own zones, punching in whatever age adjusts the workout to your own Max HR and training zones.

Regardless of your preferred indoor activities, you'll want to get creative in order to overcome boredom. You can either invent games to play on your favorite machine or use multiple pieces of equipment to work different muscle groups. Here are some suggestions for spicing up your indoor workouts with indoor cross-training.

Five-Minute Circuits

Start by learning how to use one piece of equipment, such as a motorized treadmill, and work out on it for five minutes. When you feel comfortable with it, add a second piece to your routine, such as a stair-stepper, for another five-minute period. Work your way up to the point where you can move easily from one piece of cardiovascular equipment to the next, staying on each long enough to note its effect on your heart rate. You'll quickly realize that equipment that uses both your upper and lower body, like the rowing, skiing, and climbing machines, raises your heart rates higher than those that isolate a specific muscle group, such as the stationary bicycle.

"The weight equipment was a real eye-opener for me," said Michael. "I'm not really shy, but I could use the rowing machine and treadmill at my club without any instruction. Somehow, I'd look over at the exercise machines, but I wouldn't take the time to get someone to help me figure them out. I'm glad you talked me into taking the plunge, Sal, because my workouts on these machines have definitely increased my all-around strength."

Let me talk you into something now, too. Whatever indoor activity has attracted your curiosity—free weights, aerobic dancing, weight machines, ballroom dancing—don't let shyness keep you from joining in the fun.

Single-Zone Stations

Before doing Single-Zone Stations you need to select three to five of your favorite pieces of cardiovascular training equipment and one workout zone, such as Z3, the Aerobic zone. Perform a five-minute set on each device, staying in your predetermined workout zone, then do a second set by repeating the sequence. Use any machines you like.

Multiple-Zone Stations

Like the single-zone stations workout, you start Multiple-Zone Stations by selecting three of your favorite pieces of cardiovascular equipment. On the first piece of equipment, exercise five minutes in Z1, the Healthy Heart zone. Move to the second piece and exercise for five minutes in Z2, the Temperate zone. Move to the last piece and spend five minutes in Z3, the Aerobic zone; then repeat the series. By using different body parts and multiple zones you'll get multiple benefits from this efficient workout plan. Michael uses the treadmill for Z1, the rowing machine for Z2, and the stair-stepper for Z3. You could use that plan or come up with your own.

Preprogrammed Workouts

Most of the more sophisticated exercise machines offer preprogrammed workouts, which you select by entering certain information, such as time and difficulty level. Try out these programs to see which you enjoy most, then use the creativity of the equipment manufacturer to set your workout. For example, a rowing machine may ask if you want to compete against another rower on the screen. Go for it! A little competition can add some fun to your workout. "My friend Bing and I play this little game," says Michael. "We get so bored on the treadmills, we set up a three-mile race as we run side by side. That trick keeps our boredom at bay."

Work, Work, Work

Although I championed the concept of cross-training more than a decade ago, I can't take credit for its tremendous popularity these days. It has gained favor, I suspect, not only because it delivers so many benefits to all-around fitness but because multiple-sport workouts add so much fun to the fitness equation. For many of us, the outdoors is a gym full of workout activities where we trade the fixed rowing machines, treadmills, and aerobics studios for free space, fresh air, and sunlight. The outdoors is a place where anyone can have fun while getting or staying in shape.

You can add to your Heart Zone Training points by working outdoors, not just working out outdoors. I'm talking about real physical work. Let's say you live in an area where it snows. Shoveling snow may be a necessity, but why hire someone else to do it for you? Why not, like Michael, consider your shoveling time as a superb workout? Any physical labor outdoors can be a form of outdoor cross training.

How would you calculate Heart Zone Training points? Simply determine the amount of time that you want to work in your zones, then start shoveling. Measure your time-in-zone, and when the snow's all shoveled, add the workout to your log. It's just as valuable as any other workout. Give physical work exercise credit and points.

Work is work. Make no distinction between exercise work and physical labor work. The body doesn't know the difference—it only knows that for improved health, fitness, and performance, it must sustain the "work" in different zones. It doesn't discriminate among working out on a rowing a machine, rowing a boat, or plowing a row. It only knows workload—your heart rate during large-muscle use multiplied by the amount of time spent in-zone.

What if you need to clean your house on workout day? Again, your body doesn't care whether you mop the floor or go to a club for an aerobics class. So why not build heart zone cleaning (sweeping, vacuuming, scrubbing, or whatever) into your exercise routine? Record your efforts according to the zone and the amount of time-in-zone. If you want to clean in Z3, the Aerobic zone, then you simply have to work at a higher intensity level when you are vacuuming or shoveling snow.

I know my neighbors must chuckle when they watch me doing yard work. I run while pushing an old-fashioned manual lawn mower, but that effort keeps me in my Aerobic zone. When it's time to empty the bag of grass clippings, I take my rest interval. I enjoy mowing the lawn because I earn Heart Zone Training points!

Another kind of outdoor cross-training includes putting together the four components of total fitness (coordination skills, cardiovascular conditioning, strength training, and range of motion or flexibility) during the same workout. You can easily do this by using an established par course or making one of your own. The next time you engage in Heart Zone Training, which is mostly cardiovascular conditioning, allow yourself to interrupt the session to do a few push-ups and sit-ups, stretch during a water break, or work on coordination skills that require balance.

You don't have to keep your heart rate in the same zone throughout the session. Since fitness benefits accumulate, allow yourself recuperation time for other activities, then take off and resume your cardiovascular conditioning. A little variety adds more fun, and it even gives you more benefit in less time. When I see runners run in place when forced to stop at a traffic light, I say to myself that they should stop, rest, and let their heart rates drop. If they did, they would be gaining the benefits of interval training.

When I suggested to Michael that he set up his own par course in his front yard, he responded with the usual enthusiasm. When spring rolled around, he put on his sweat suit and selected his workout equipment: a rake, a shovel, an ax, a maul, a wheelbarrow, a tennis ball, and his dog Holly. Then he laid out his course: the garden, the wood pile, and the grassy area where Holly loved to retrieve her ball.

"I said, okay, here's my gym. First I raked up the fallen leaves and carted them to the compost heap (twenty minutes, including ten minutes in my Z3 Aerobic zone at 114 to 130 bpm and ten minutes in Z1). Then I tossed the ball and chased Holly (five minutes, during which my heart rate zoomed all the way up to my Z4 Threshold zone of 130 to 146 bpm). More ball-tossing for Holly got me down to my Z2 Temperate zone (fifteen minutes, during which my heart rate settled at 98 to 114 bpm), lower this time."

Michael's total Heart Zone Training points?

Raking leaves:	10 minutes x Z3 = 30 points;
More raking leaves:	10 minutes x Z1 = 10 points;
Tossing and chasing:	5 minutes x Z4 = 20 points;
More tossing:	15 minutes x Z2 = 30 points

A grand total of ninety Heart Zone Training points. For Michael, that's enough multiple-zone exercise for his total workout for the day.

"That's a good hour at the club," he laughed. "But what a ball Holly and I had turning our front yard into a gym."

Which Workouts Are the Best?

Many questions still go unanswered in the world of fitness. Which is better for you, thirty minutes of tennis or thirty minutes of racquetball? Does thirty minutes of one offer the same fitness value as thirty minutes of the other? You may ask yourself, "Do I get better conditioning from riding an exercise bike for fifteen minutes or cycling on the road bike for fifteen minutes?" Or you may wonder whether it's better to play eighteen holes of golf carrying your bag or to walk the same distance carrying the same weight but not making stops to hit a ball?

Researchers have been seeking answers to these kinds of questions for years. Typically, sports scientists hook up study participants to assessment devices that can measure how many calories of energy their bodies are expending or how much oxygen they take in when performing different activities.

After nearly fifty years of research, almost unanimous agreement has arisen that exercise benefits result less from a given exercise or sport than from fitness programs that exercise your large muscles, resulting in cardiovascular benefits, strength building, and flexibility or range of motion. You can do this indoors. You can do it outdoors. You can do it working or playing continuously, with intervals or with rest periods. You can do it alone or with a group. You can do it with a racquet in your hand or a golf bag on your shoulder.

The key to your optimum all-around fitness depends on comparing the different activities in which you participate by using the Heart Zone Training point system described in the previous chapter. The chart below compares the values of different exercises. Keep in mind that you can engage in the same activity in different zones by increasing or reducing workload.

Getting Creative with Your Fitness Program

TYPICAL ACTIVITIES AND THEIR POINT VALUES

ACTIVITY	ZONE NUMBER	TIME	TOTAL HZT POINTS
Tennis	Z3	15 minutes	45 points
Shoveling	Z4	10 minutes	40 points
Walking	Z1	50 minutes	50 points
Vacuuming	Z2	25 minutes	50 points
Bicycling	Z5	8 minutes	40 points
Swimming	Z1	45 minutes	45 points
Basketball	Z3	15 minutes	45 points
Making Love	Z1	15 minutes	15 points
Dance Aerobics	Z3	15 minutes	45 points

As you can see, one activity is not intrinsically better than another. Sure, cycling strengthens the leg muscles more than swimming, but does that make cycling better than swimming? It's better than swimming for the leg muscles, but swimming is better than cycling for the arm muscles. In your case, will forty-five Heart Zone Training points of playing tennis benefit you more than forty-five Heart Zone Training points of playing basketball? The answer is that both of these sports activities are better at strengthening, sharpening and improving certain parts and systems of the body than other sports activities.

That's why you should incorporate cross-training into your all-around fitness program. If you decide that you love to walk and that's the only activity you're going to do, you will get fit, I guarantee it. But you will only get "walk fit," not "totally fit." Walk fit may be just fine for you; but on the other hand, for the same amount of time, energy, and cost, you can get totally fit by adding multi-activity conditioning or cross-training to your program.

Every personal Heart Zone Training program should incorporate variety and creativity. Earn as many Heart Zone Training points as you want, but obtain them in a variety of ways in order to achieve all-around fitness. The best road to fitness for anyone does what Michael's did for him: It keeps you traveling down a path full of surprises and enjoyment.

Sex

As long as we are on the topic of creative Heart Zone Training, I'd like to dispel one more myth—the myth of sex as exercise. If you find yourself in a cardiac rehabilitation program, sex can be a little scary. In fact, any increase in heart rate can cause some fear or anxiety over the potential risk involved. So what does happen to your heart rate during sexual activity?

The fact is, we know more about the effects of exercise on athletes and astronauts than we know about the effects of sexual exercise on people in their bedrooms. Even less information is available about the sexual activity of people who have experienced heart disease. It's difficult to study human and sexual activity without running into all kinds of obstacles—psychological, physiological, and ethical.

Nevertheless, research published to date in major medical journals gives us some answers. According to these reports, the average heart rate for men in the "on top" position hits 117 bpm for about ten to twenty seconds of peak experience, orgasm. Women average around 100 beats per minute during that brief period.

These numbers may seem surprisingly low, but the truth is, sex really isn't all that strenuous. The large muscle groups involved in, say, running or cross country skiing simply do not come into play. Most of the work is done by the abdominal and smaller muscles, and since most people make love in a horizontal rather than a vertical position, the heart rate numbers drop even further. The period of high activity and excitement is so brief, only ten to twenty seconds at peak time, that you really can't earn a lot of Heart Zone Training points from making love.

Of course, individuals differ greatly. Age and familiarity play an important role in determining workload during sex. But if you were disappointed to read that lovemaking is not great Heart Zone Training, you may be reassured to find out that studies also show a very low incidence of death related to coitus at home with one's spouse or partner. (The death rates do run higher if the two individuals are not familiar with each other.) One Japanese researcher, for example, reported that of 5,559 sudden deaths studied, less than 1 percent, or a total of thirty-four people, died during sexual activity. The conclusion from this and other research is that from a strictly cardiovascular viewpoint, sex does not appear to pose a high risk for the majority of the population.

Sexual activity does, however, provide a Z1 Healthy Heart zone workout. Rarely will it reach into the Z2 Temperate zone, even though a person might perceive himself or herself to be Z5 redlining. You can always slip on a heart rate monitor and check for yourself. If you wish to fulfill the ACSM (American College of Sports Medicine) guidelines for minimum exercise intensity and workout time, you'll be disappointed. Sexual workouts won't qualify.

Challenging Your Creativity

Let your mind run aerobically wild for a moment and ask yourself, "What would I love to accomplish?" What finish banner could you cross under and feel that surge of self-satisfaction when taking the last step, pedaling the final meter, or swimming the last stroke? Fix that dream firmly in mind as I recount a recent experience.

Last year I finished dead last in every Danskin Women's Triathlon Series event. That's right, dead last, me, an accomplished runner. How did that happen? Well, my job was not to win the race but to support, encourage, cajole, and sometimes act like a devil with a poker in my hand as I prodded every woman to finish no matter how tired or beat up she felt. As I brought in the last swimmer, she was always swimming the backstroke—her best but always the slowest stroke. The final swimmer usually passes the last biker riding a bike that has been hanging in the garage for the past ten years. The final bike finisher generally catches and passes the final runner-walker.

This year, as I approached the last runner, she hollered at me without turning back to look, "I hear you catching me, Sally!" Sure enough, it was the same woman who finished last in the race held the year before, but this time our journey to the finish line was different. The previous year, Susan Thompson told me her story; about the Fulbright scholarship she had earned and an auto accident soon after that had caused brain damage and put her into a coma for nearly six months. Susan had come out of her coma knowing neither her name nor her past. She had had to start from scratch, learning to read and speak again—finding out who she was.

This year, as I started to walk those last few miles in the triathlon with Susan, she said, "Sal, I am in better shape, and you can tell. I'm closer to the finish line than when you caught me last year. I spent the whole year training just so I could tell you that when you caught me. I knew I would be last, but I promised myself I would be further and faster, and I am. I read your book and trained with a heart rate monitor and I want to tell you, this race is my mountain top."

Susan told me that each year she selects a physical challenge difficult for her to imagine. This year that challenge was to finish the triathlon race faster than she had the year before. When we crossed that finish line, her friends were there to cheer and celebrate her victory of finishing *second to last*. At the end, the two of us looked at each other. Susan was smiling, sweaty and exhausted, but she knew in her heart that she had reached the top of her personal mountain. The feeling that makes a person who she is, confident, committed, and complete, was all hers. She had *earned* that feeling.

What greater reward can you give yourself than the challenge of a physical test, whether it's a triathlon or your first one-mile walk or a one-hundred-mile bike ride? Heart Zone Training bestows that reward, creating the sort of lifestyle change that empowers you to become everything you can be. It bestows a healthy life full of heart and full of purpose. It all starts with the physical, the body, and getting it healthy.

You can challenge yourself in many ways. I like to write down all of the different events I might enter on slips of paper. I spread the pieces of paper out on a table and write the dates of the different events on each. Then I shuffle the papers, trying to put them into some kind of priority order. After I add the events on the top several papers to my planning calendar, I begin the process of training and accomplishing them. As I do this I always ask myself, "Is it realistic to accomplish this challenge, given the other factors and events in my life?"

Big successes begin with small steps. The Japanese call it *kaizen*—"constant small improvements." They understand that if you improve yourself 1 percent 100 times, you will realize a 100-percent lifestyle change. We westerners tend to think you have to improve 100 percent one time, but to become a competitive athlete, I started by running one mile, then adding a mile, then adding another mile. Those constant small improvements led to 100-mile ultra marathons. The rewards along the way were frequent, and the lifestyle change was permanent.

So I challenge you to challenge your own fitness creativity. Join an athletic club and make an agreement to work out there four times a week. Sign up for a class to learn a new sport. Set aside a date to enter an athletic competition, and start training. Learn to play tennis, enlist a friend to become your doubles partner to keep you on the court. Cross-train indoors and outdoors. By accomplishing your challenge, you will feel a sense of exhilaration beyond your wildest dreams.

Your Personal Challenge Log

Try to come up with ten challenges, ranging from those you know you can accomplish fairly easily—such as running a mile or losing five pounds or starting a weight-training program—to those that may seem almost impossible at this point in your training—such as running a marathon or losing fifty pounds or bench pressing two hundred pounds. Set a target, reset it whenever necessary, and record your accomplishments as they take place.

CHALLENGE	TARGET DATE	ACTUAL DATE
1.		
2.		
3.		
4.		
5.		
6.		
7.		
8.		
9.		
10.		

Reaching the Most Advanced
Level of Heart Zone Training

Do you belong to a running club?

Are you training for a marathon?

Do you think of yourself as a serious competitor in basketball, tennis, swimming, rowing, racquetball, or any other strenuous sport?

Are you a dedicated runner, triathlete, or bodybuilder?

Do you spend eight or more hours a week working out in a health club or gym?

Have you achieved a level of optimum fitness?

Do you want to make the transition from recreational, fitness-oriented athlete to earnest competitor?

If you answer yes to any of these questions, then you're ready for this chapter, which takes Heart Zone Training to the most advanced level. If, on the other hand, you are getting all the benefits you desire from exercising regularly in the Healthy Heart, Temperate, and Aerobic zones, then you may want to skip ahead to the final chapter. High-performance training is not for everyone. It's for people like fitness enthusiast and working mom Cathy Anderson-Meyers, who has set her sights on competing in, and winning, a triathlon.

Cathy just turned forty. Though she's a busy woman, as a mother with two young children who operates her own home-based snowshoe touring business, she has maintained a rigorous exercise program for all the years I've known her. Why, I wondered, had she never tried a triathlon? When I suggested to her that she consider training for and entering her first triathlon, she loved the idea. With an important race coming up in three months, she asked me to help her plan a twelve-week training program that would get her in top form. Her busy schedule allowed thirty minutes a day for the program, so we divided that time into a six-workout week of two swims, two bike rides, and two runs.

Three months later, after nearly fifteen years of not participating in competitive sports, Cathy stood at the triathlon starting line with her number one cheerleader, her husband, watching from the sidelines, and 1,000 other women racers, her ardent supporters. She finished the race in one hour and thirty-five minutes and walked out to meet me on the course as I was running/walking in with the final finisher. Exuberant and bursting with energy, she gave me a high five and shouted, "Sally, I love it! I want more!"

I've written this chapter for those who want more. I've also written it for competitors like Bob Crowley, a long-time runner dedicated to learning how far he can push his body. Bob asked me to help him train for the Western States 100-Mile Endurance Run held each June. He trusts me because I won the race several years before. Since he had competed in dozens of marathons, he knew what it took to participate in an endurance contest, but he knew nothing yet about Heart Zone Training. I taught him about steady-state heart rate intervals, about training at his threshold heart rate, and about measuring and monitoring his workouts. Like Cathy, he fell in love with the program when he saw how much Heart Zone Training could improve his training and racing performance. After one preliminary fifty-mile race in preparation for the big event, he said, "Sally, I ran one and a half hours faster and more easily than last year. I wasn't exhausted at the finish line because I followed your highest sustainable Max HR system and used a monitor. It worked."

Higher performance training starts with four concepts:

- Maximum heart rate
- Training tree
- Time-in-zone
- HZT point system

Determining Your Zone Anchor Point

Your Max HR provides the anchor point around which you set all five of your heart zones. Your Max HR is a specific number—the maximum number of contractions that your heart can make per minute. Take a moment to review the basic facts about Max HR in Chapter 1. You'll need this crucial piece of information, because you will be designing your advanced Heart Zone Training program around it.

Keep one additional point in mind. Max HR is sport-specific, so if you train in different sports, you must allocate different zone ranges for each activity. For example, my Max HR when running is 200 bpm, but my Max HR when swimming is only 175 bpm. I must adjust my zones when I train in these different disciplines.

Climbing the Training Tree

In Chapter 5 you learned about the six branches of the training tree. As your level of fitness rises, you move up the branches to the top, and as you recover, you drop down to the trunk and go easy, consciously resting during your workout sessions. Keeping track of your Time-In-Zone (TIZ) encourages you to increase the amount of time you spend on those higher branches as a percentage of your total workout time, and the Heart Zone Training Point System enables you to quantify total workload by multiplying the zone number by the number of minutes in that zone.

The high-performance or competitive athlete trains heavily on the upper branches of the tree, setting TIZ according to a specific goal. Pick a race, a tournament, or an event, then determine the number of weeks available for training. Since successful competitors train gradually, you will want to set aside a sufficient number of weeks for your own training, usually four to eight weeks. Use the Heart Zone Training Points Log introduced in Chapter 5 to develop your advanced Heart Zone Training program, planning specific workouts with built-in progressions.

Designing your Time-In-Zone Training Program

Let's see how Cathy Anderson-Meyers used TIZ to plan her training for her second triathlon. First of all, she set aside a

full twelve weeks for her training, because this event represented a big challenge for her, even though she was in very
good shape. Her specific goal was to complete the international distance triathlon, which consists of a 1.5K swim, 40K
bike, and 10K run (1-mile swim, 25-mile bike, 6.2-mile run)
in under three hours. For each of the twelve weeks she
decided to commit seven hours a week, or one hour per day,
to exercise. That meant a typical workout might range from
forty-five to ninety minutes. Cathy started on the interval
branch because that's where she felt comfortable at the
beginning of her training.

Because Max HR is sports-specific, Cathy began by
testing herself and setting her Max HR in each of the three
sports of triathlon—swimming, biking, and running. Then
she set her zones based on percentages of those numbers.
She found the following results:

MAXIMUM HEART RATE AND ZONES BY SPORT

ZONE PERCENTAGES	ZONE NUMBER	MAX HR: SWIM 180 BPM	MAX HR: BIKE 190 BPM	MAX HR: RUN 200 BPM
90%–100%	Z5	162–180	171–190	180–200
80%–90%	Z4	144–162	152–171	160–180
70%–80%	Z3	126–144	133–152	140–160
60%–70%	Z2	108–126	114–133	120–140
50%–60%	Z1	90–108	95–114	100–120

She then wrote a Heart Zone Training workout schedule
matching the amount of time (one hour a day) that she had
available and the branch of the training tree she was currently training on.

Sally Edwards' Heart Zone Training

CATHY'S HZT PLAN FOR THE TRIATHLON

BRANCH: Interval Branch

GOAL: Break 3 hours in an international distance triathlon 12 weeks from today.

DAILY AVERAGE TIME: 60 minutes

RANGE: 45–90 minutes per day

DAY	TIME	ZONE	ZONE NUMBER	HR ZONE	TYPE
MONDAY	60 minutes	Aerobic	Z3	140–160	Continuous run at 150 bpm Stretching for 1/2 hour
TUESDAY	15 minutes 15 minutes	Redline Temperate	Z5 Z2	180–200 120–140	Bike: 3 x 5 minutes at 175 Rest intervals 3 x 5 minutes at 120
WEDNESDAY	60 minutes	Temperate	Z2	120–140	Recovery run: slow and easy
THURSDAY	60 minutes	Threshold	Z4	145–160	Swim intervals
FRIDAY	60 minutes	Aerobic	Z3	140–150	Brick: Run 20 minutes/Bike 40
SATURDAY	45 minutes	Threshold	Z4	145–150	Continuous swim at highest sustainable heart rate pace
SUNDAY	90 minutes	Aerobic	Z3	140–150	Long bike ride

Reaching the Most Advanced Level of Heart Zone Training

CATHY'S HZT POINTS LOG

	MONTH/DATE	SPORT ACTIVITY	Z1	Z2	Z3	Z4	Z5	TOTAL POINTS	DAILY NOTES	COMMENTS
					TIME IN ZONES					
MONDAY	5/10	Run			60			180	Resting HR: 62 Weight: 155 Other:	Easy Day
TUESDAY	5/11	Bike		15			15	105	Resting HR: Weight: 154 Other:	
WEDNESDAY	5/12	Run		60				120	Resting HR: 61 Weight: 154 Other:	
THURSDAY	5/13	Swim			60	60		240	Resting HR: 62 Weight: 153 Other:	
FRIDAY	5/14	Run Bike			60			180	Resting HR: 61 Weight: 153 Other:	
SATURDAY	5/15	Swim						180	Resting HR: 62 Weight: 153 Other:	
SUNDAY	5/16	Bike			90			270	Resting HR: 62 Weight: 154 Other:	
			Z1	75	210	60	15	1275	WEEKLY HZT POINTS TOTAL	
				Z2	Z3	Z4	Z5			
				19%	64%	14%	3%		% TIZ	

Total Weekly HZT Points: Multiply the time in each zone by the number of that zone.

ZONE NAME	ZONE POINTS	% OF MAX HR
Redline Zone	5	100–90%
Threshold Zone	4	90–80%
Aerobic Zone	3	80–70%
Temperate Zone	2	70–60%
Healthy Heart Zone	1	60–50%

This plan tells Cathy exactly what workout to do on any given day: what sport, for how long, and in what zone. A well-organized person by nature, she appreciates the value of budgeting her workout time and maximizing the benefits she gains from every minute of her training program. This kind of organization takes time to prepare, but it pays off handsomely for the serious competitor.

Cathy shaped her weekly training schedule by determining the amount of time available in minutes and dividing that total among the appropriate training tree branches. As you can see from her Heart Zone Training Points Log, she spent 83 percent of her time in Z2 and Z3 and 17 percent of her time in Z4 and Z5. Depending on your own current limb, you may need to adjust your workouts according to the specific sport and your goal event. Remember the training tree in Chapter 5? Cathy is on the Interval branch, which means she will spend 10 percent of her time in Z2, 60 percent of her time in Z3; 10 percent of her time in Z4, and 10 percent of her time in Z5 (Redline). Cathy knows she has 420 minutes, and she divides them up as she did in the chart below based on how much time she plans to spend in each zone during her week:

PERCENTAGE OF TIZ
BRANCH: Interval

ZONE NUMBER	TIZ PERCENTAGE	TIZ MINUTES
Z5	10%	42 minutes
Z4	10%	84 minutes
Z3	60%	252 minutes
Z2	20%	42 minutes
Z1		

This planning method allocates the number of minutes you will work out each week in the various training tree branches. It also provides you proper progressive adaptation, enabling you to spend the same amount of time and get progressively more benefits from your training workload by allowing you to climb up the training tree and spend more time in higher zones.

Many serious athletes add training time to their plans as they move up the tree, gaining even more points. Others gain more points by adding more time in the higher zones rather than by increasing total training time. It all depends on your schedule.

If you miss a workout or even a few in a row, don't make the mistake of trying to make them up all at once. Overtraining can hurt your performance as much as undertraining. We all miss workouts from time to time, and that's okay. You don't have to make up the points at all. You simply need to adjust your training schedule appropriately. If it doesn't fit your particular lifestyle, design a new schedule that does. All busy people struggle to juggle their limited time, but there's always a way to come up with a Heart Zone Training program that works, if you plan your workout schedule carefully.

There are lots of tricks to increasing your available training time. You can get up earlier, work out during eating periods, eat during workout periods, or combine social and workout time by inviting your friends and partners to train with you. Make your training tree and your time-in-zone an integral part of your lifestyle. Make it fit into, not around, your life.

By using Heart Zone Training points you can measure and "reward" yourself for performance. All competitors relish rewards, and they tend to establish their own individual systems. After all, individuals differ in the amount of workload or FIT they can tolerate and still remain healthy. If you've been training for dozens of years, your tolerance levels for exercise intensity and time-in-zone will be higher than those of novice athletes.

Don't Overtrain

It's important to remember that when some athletes' points exceed a certain number, deconditioning sets in and they actually get less fit. Overtraining results in a loss of aerobic fitness, which is one of the forms of deconditioning. When you train too long at a time in the upper two zones, Threshold and Redline, you can stress your system beyond its ability to repair and rebuild.

Beyond a certain workload, the body can't adequately rebuild and maintain itself. Those who overtrain to the point of deconditioning frequently suffer from colds, respiratory difficulties, and immune system problems. They suffer chronic fatigue, they lack energy, they even injure themselves. Physical breakdown affects overtrained competitors every day; be sure you never make that mistake.

From a research perspective, it's not clear how many Heart Zone Training points a person can earn before overtraining occurs. However, according to Dr. Carl Foster, exercise physiologist at the Milwaukee Heart Institute, "Olympic ice skaters seem to be able to handle about 6,000 weekly Heart Zone Training points during their peak performance period, while participatory athletes like me can only tolerate about 2,000 points before they become stale, and beginners start with 100 points." It's up to you to determine what workload your body can safely handle throughout your training schedule.

Getting Down to Training Essentials

For the competitive athlete, interval training and training in multiple and higher zones is essential. Alternating work intervals with rest/recovery intervals is the key to getting faster and moving your anaerobic threshold closer to your Max HR. Trainers usually express the relationship between the two intervals as a ratio. For example, if you bike at a Z5 steady-state heart rate for five minutes and then actively rest at a Z2 heart rate for five minutes, the work-to-recovery interval ratio is 1:1 (five minutes of work and five minutes of recovery).

Note how these numbers differ from the Heart Zone Training points you earn. If you spend five minutes in Z5, you earn twenty-five points, but if you spend five minutes in Z2, you only earn ten points. It's important to know that both Z5 points and Z2 points as in this example are important. You need to stress your anaerobic system by being in the top zones and you need to allow it recovery time by being in the lower zones. That's an essential concept.

As for the ratio, there is no one right ratio. At first you will discover you need more active rest time to high-intensity time, so your ratio will be something like 1:3, or one time increment in Z4 or Z5 to three time increments in Z1 or Z2. As you get fitter you will become comfortable with a 1:2 and eventually a 1:1 ratio, while for elite athletes, the high-intensity time becomes the bigger side of the ratio, with workloads of 2:1 and 4:1 common. That's because once the body has adapted to this overload of exercise, it can recover more quickly and be ready for the next bout.

Another way to classify intervals is by total time spent in each. During short burst intervals you may go all out for ten to twenty seconds at top speed and near your Max HR. During middle, long, and endurance intervals, you may go twenty seconds to ten minutes at a slower speed and at a lower HR. In general, when you train at higher and higher heart rate levels, the intervals become shorter.

During longer intervals you are training your body's different energy expenditure systems to deliver different amounts and kinds of energy. When exercising in Z5, for example, your energy delivery system burns a high quantity of carbohydrates at high rates of burning, much like a solid-fueled rocket engine, as compared to a liquid-fuel engine. When you train in Z1, the Healthy Heart zone, you are burning a very low percentage of carbohydrates but higher amounts of fat calories. When you are burning fat, you are not training your fuel system to burn what it needs for high-performance expenditure. When you are burning carbohydrates at high-intensity Z4 and Z5 zones, you are not training your fuel system to burn fat as a source of energy. The most successful athletic competitors maintain the right ratio of fuels as they burn them. By training and racing too long in a too-high zone, you can deplete your glycogen, or muscle carbohydrate fuel sources and end up virtually running out of gas.

What's the right blend of fuels? Well, it depends on your current conditioning, your nutritional program, and your zone. If you are really, really fit, you can burn a lot of fat as fuel at high zones because your anaerobic threshold heart rate is so high you don't break out of fat metabolism until you are at really, really high heart rates. That's why athletes are such good fat burners; they have trained their fuel system to burn huge quantities of fat.

For me, a common Heart Zone interval training session involves running one-mile repetitions, each of which pushes me higher up the training tree. For the first mile I start at my Z2 floor and take myself up to the midpoint of my Z4. This takes me about six minutes and ten seconds. I then recover a bit by jogging 1/4 mile. During the next mile I take my heart five beats higher than the mile before, clocking about a six-minute mile. After another recovering jog, I do another five beats higher, finishing that mile in around five minutes and fifty seconds. Another recovery and I run the last "killer" interval. I hold that interval at yet another five beats higher until the last 1/4-mile, when I "redline," zooming up to 95 percent of my Max HR. I can barely hold that intensity for the final 1/4-mile stretch. My legs hurt, and my breathing is rapid and deep. Finally I jog, then walk during a ten-minute warm-down, and end the session. What do I gain from this ladder interval? I get faster. You will, too, if you take the key training principles to heart.

Embracing the Five Key Training Principles

Throughout this book I've repeatedly stressed the need for Heart Zone Trainers to monitor their heart rates and measure their progress toward targeted goals. This applies especially to the serious athlete. The tools you've learned to use in this book take the guesswork out of training for competition. If you really want to perform at your personal best, then you should apply all the Heart Zone Training tools to these five key training principles.

Principle 1: Train At, About, or Around Your Anaerobic Threshold Heart Rate

At your Z4 Threshold zone your heart rate will reach between 80 and 90 percent of your Max HR. Most people who have undergone scientific testing find that their Anaerobic Threshold heart rate point (ATHR) does indeed land somewhere in that range, where your body crosses over the threshold from aerobic to anaerobic metabolism. At the floor of the zone the body usually has sufficient oxygen to meet the demands of a high level of exercise intensity. However, when you increase workload beyond your ATHR, you move into an anaerobic state where your body cannot supply enough oxygen to meet your muscles' demands. Scientists also measure this state in terms of lactate levels in the blood; this is called the lactate threshold. Some measure ATHR with a respirator gas analyzer, which measures the amount of gas you exchange. This method provides you with your VO_2 anaerobic threshold. Both of these threshold points are usually about the same heart rate number.

Your anaerobic threshold heart rate point changes with conditioning. As you become fitter, it goes up; as you lose fitness, it goes down. Serious athletes push to raise their anaerobic threshold heart rate point as close as possible to their Max HR. This is the true definition of aerobic, cardio-vascular fitness. For example, when I am not training for competition, my ATHR might fall to around 160 bpm, but when I heart zone train for a race, it can rise as high as 185 bpm. That twenty-five-point increase indicates that my body has adapted to strenuous exercise and can deliver more oxygen, performing more effectively.

The key to getting faster lies in training at your ATHR, moving it as close as possible to your Max HR. To raise your ATHR, you must train at, about, or, around that specific number. If, for example, I want to raise my ATHR higher than 160 bpm, I need to spend a lot of time training in a zone around that heart rate number. If I spend too much time training above it, I will be overtraining and incurring the setbacks of deconditioning; if I spend too much time training below it, I will stay fit but I will not get fitter.

To measure your ATHR accurately, you must have yourself tested in a sports science lab, hospital, or other facility where specialists can precisely determine oxygen or lactate levels. However, you can make a fairly accurate "guesstimate" with the "Dave Martin Two Times Twenty Minutes" test. Select a sport activity and go as hard as you can for twenty minutes. Record your average heart rate for that time, then rest for five minutes. Go for another hard twenty minutes and again record your average heart rate. The average heart rate of both twenty-minute periods represents a fairly accurate ATHR number. This extremely strenuous workout will tire you, so prepare yourself for that feeling. Do *not* take this test unless you are in excellent shape and feel comfortable exercising extremely hard for forty minutes.

Principles 2: Train at Maximum Sustainable and Steady-State Heart Rates

You can measure your training progress in a number of different ways, but I prefer using maximum sustainable heart rate and steady-state heart rates. Your maximum sustainable heart rate is the highest heart rate number you can sustain over a given distance. The higher the number, the faster you will finish the event. As your anaerobic threshold heart rate goes higher during dedicated Heart Zone Training, your maximum sustainable heart rate will naturally rise. Of course, your maximum sustainable heart rate will go down in proportion to the length of a race or event. In a marathon, for example, I can only sustain 172 bpm, but in a 10K (6.2-mile) running race I can sustain 183 bpm.

Competitors frequently use steady-state heart rates for self-tests or time trials. Find a measured course, such as a three-mile bike path, and set your heart rate goal at a steady state number such as 155 bpm. Warmup, then start the test when you reach 155 bpm. Try to stay within one or two beats of that number for the entire three miles, then measure the elapsed time. As you get fitter, the time will shorten.

Steady-state heart rates also work nicely during workout ladders. One of my favorite swim workouts involves 300-yard repeats at different ascending steady-state heart rates. I swim my first 300 yards at a steady-state 125 bpm, then I increase each repeat by five-beat increments until I reach 150 bpm.

Principle 3: Watch for Cardiac Drift

If you train or race for long distances or long periods of time, your heart rate will gradually float upward, even though you are going at the same speed. This phenomenon, known as cardiac drift, occurs mostly as the result of dehydration. In very simple terms, as you lose the fluid in your body, your heart must work harder and beat faster to supply the muscles with the same amount of blood.

By watching for cardiac drift, you can monitor changes in your body when training or racing. If you haven't been drinking enough fluids and your heart rate starts drifting, you know it's time to begin drinking. If cardiac drift occurs when you have been consuming fluids, you should re-evaluate the quantity, quality, or timing of your fluid intake.

Ultimately, everyone who trains or races beyond a certain distance will experience cardiac drift regardless of how much fluid they drink. Stay well hydrated to keep cardiac drift to a minimum, and your performance will remain at the highest possible level.

Principle 4: Observe the 10-percent and 50-percent Rules

I must confess that, like a lot of serious athletes, I have developed a lactic acid addiction. Those of us with this addiction love to work out in the Z5 Redline zone, going as hard and as fast as possible. Workouts in Z1 or Z2 don't excite us much, and we struggle to stay below the ceilings of those zones. That's why serious athletes need some rules. Otherwise we'd pursue an exclusive lactic acid training program with far too little time devoted to recovery and rebuilding.

The 10-percent rule states that no single workout in Threshold (Z4) or Redline (Z5) can exceed more than 10 percent of the week's total time. In other words, if you are going to train 420 minutes per week, spend no more than 42 minutes of any one training session at Z4 or Z5.

The 50-percent rule states that you can spend no more than 50 percent of the week's total training time in the Threshold (Z4) and Redline (Z5) zones. These zones are the "hot zones"; if you spend too much time in them, you risk the negative effects of overtraining. For the high-performance endurance athlete who knows the importance of long intervals at high sustainable heart rates, it's easy to train too hard and too long. By using Heart Zone Training and recording your time-in-zone, you can measure and control your training so that it enhances rather than undermines your performance.

Principle 5: Obey the Twenty-Four-Hour and Forty-Eight-Hour Rules

Two practical rules apply to both the single-sport athlete and the multi-sport participant. The twenty-four-hour rule states that you can do one Z5 Redline zone workout every twenty-four hours, provided you change activities the next day. It's OK to swim in Z5 one day, bike in Z5 the next and cross country ski in Z5 the day after that. By changing sports, you change muscle groups, thus allowing your sport-specific muscles to rest and recover before the next Z4 or Z5 workout.

The forty-eight-hour rule relates to a single sport. It states that you must wait forty-eight hours before doing another Z5 or Z4 workout in the same sport. If you run in Z5 on Monday, you can run in Z4 or Z5 on Wednesday, provided you rest on Tuesday. During these forty-eight hours of rest, the specific muscles you used gain sufficient time to recover. It takes the body at least forty-eight hours to replenish the fuel stores necessary to sustain another high-zone workout.

Forging the Mind and Body Connection

For the first time in the history of fitness and sports, a training system provides us with a tool that links our minds and our bodies. Serious athletes have begun to use the heart rate monitor religiously, and not just during their workouts. The monitor is one piece of equipment anyone can buy. When the heart responds to increased exercise intensity by beating faster, the monitor relays that information instantly to the mind. The mind can then process the information and respond to the heart's message by going easier, staying steady, or picking up the intensity.

- Heart rate monitoring generates useful biofeedback.
- Heart rate monitoring enables optimum fitness training.
- Heart rate monitoring teaches about stress.
- Heart rate monitoring helps burn fat calories.
- Heart rate monitoring wins races.

I always race by heart rate, not pace. When running by pace or minutes per mile, I cannot possibly account for physical, emotional, and environmental conditions such as uphills (or downhills), heat, humidity, and state of health. A heart rate monitoring plan takes all of these factors into account and tells you precisely how your body is responding on a particular day to that day's particular circumstances. That's why they call heart rate monitors personal power tools.

Sally Edwards' Heart Zone Training

Your Personal Log (Heart Zone Training Points Log)

MONTH/ DATE	SPORT ACTIVITY	TIME IN ZONES					TOTAL POINTS	DAILY NOTES	COMMENTS
		Z1	Z2	Z3	Z4	Z5			
MONDAY								Resting HR: Weight: Other:	
TUESDAY								Resting HR: Weight: Other:	
WEDNESDAY								Resting HR: Weight: Other:	
THURSDAY								Resting HR: Weight: Other:	
FRIDAY								Resting HR: Weight: Other:	
SATURDAY								Resting HR: Weight: Other:	
SUNDAY								Resting HR: Weight: Other:	

ZONE NAME	ZONE POINTS	% OF MAX HR
Redline Zone	5	100–90%
Threshold Zone	4	90–80%
Aerobic Zone	3	80–70%
Temperate Zone	2	70–60%
Healthy Heart Zone	1	60–50%

WEEKLY HZT POINTS TOTAL

Z1	Z2	Z3	Z4	Z5
% TIZ				

Total Weekly HZT Points: Multiply the time in each zone by the number of that zone.

Training Every Heart and Body

Real estate developer Ed Oswalt, who works on Cape Cod, has altered the old saying about the three most important variables in selling property ("location, location, location") to "water view, water view, water view." When I started him on the journey to fitness by giving him a heart rate monitor for his birthday, I told him, "Ed, your training program should include these three important variables, "the individual, the individual, the individual."

A bit sedentary and about fifteen pounds overweight, fifty-six-year-old Ed had never thought about training for anything until his doctor told him he'd feel better and look better if he added some regular aerobic exercising to his frequent walks through the woods of Truro and Wellfleet. When he asked my advice, I suggested he buy a pair of good running shoes and try a little jogging, starting out gradually and working up to three miles three times a week.

"But, Sally," he protested, "that's so boring." Ed loves gadgets, though, and his birthday present soon captured his imagination. Within three months he was jogging nine miles a week at a moderate pace, working out sixty minutes a week on a rowing machine that had been gathering dust in his garage, and feeling and looking better than he had in years. Oh, yes, he also dropped that fifteen unwanted pounds of excess weight.

Ed's story illustrates the basic truths of Heart Zone Training. First, he accepted the fact that regular exercise provides the key to physical and mental well-being. When you look better and feel better physically, your self image and mental well-being improve automatically. Second, Ed learned that the best exercise programs revolve around individual circumstances and needs. In this book you've met almost every conceivable type of individual—the unfit, the extremely fit, the overweight and the slim, the young and the old, male and female, those with lots of time to work out and those with very hectic schedules—and you've seen how each tailored a Heart Zone Training program to suit his or her particular heart, body, and lifestyle. Third, Ed understood that his program needed to add fun to his life. Whether you monitor your heart rate manually or, like Ed, use a heart rate monitor, you will enjoy getting the concrete feedback that can make your exercising not only more tangibly rewarding but also more fun.

Finally, Ed carefully followed the Ten Steps of Heart Zone Training:

THE TEN STEPS OF HEART ZONE TRAINING

1. Determine your maximum heart rate (Max HR).
2. Set your five heart training zones (Z1 through Z5).
3. Set your fitness and performance goals.
4. Pick your current training tree branch.
5. Set your weekly training time.
6. Calculate your Time-In-Zone (TIZ).
7. Determine your weekly Heart Zone Training Points.
8. Do your workouts.
9. Fill in your Heart Zone Training Points Log.
10. Complete monthly self-tests.

If you feel unsure about any of those steps, look back at the earlier chapters, especially the personal logs at the end of each chapter. For now, however, here's a quick review.

Step 1: Determine Your Maximum Heart Rate

Max HR number represents your anchor point, and it doesn't matter whether your own is a high or low number. One is not better than another. Knowing your Max HR, you can set your five zones and adjust them throughout your lifetime. As you get fitter and as you age, your heart will naturally change, and you need to take those changes into account and fine-tune your program accordingly.

Step 2: Set Your Five Heart Training Zones

Each zone from Z1 through Z5 represents 10-percent increments of your anchor point or Max HR. The five zones are progressive, with each providing a different benefit within the wellness continuum. Athletes train in different zones because they want different benefits. As you progress through the zones, you can accumulate benefits, until eventually you can earn all the benefits of training in all of the zones. Zone training applies to all sports and all physical activities. It also enriches the mind. It's a biofeedback monitor. By measuring your heart rate, you forge a strong link between your mind and your body.

Step 3: Set Your Fitness and Performance Goals

As an athlete, I have learned that the more frequently I feel a sense of accomplishment or reach my goals, the more motivated I become. That's why I set small, reachable goals and try to make frequent small fitness improvements. I don't expect gigantic leaps and changes but rather an accumulation of little improvements that add up to big ones. Goals need timelines or deadlines, and you should set specific, not general, ones.

Step 4: Pick Your Current Training Tree Branch

The training tree includes all the different levels or stages of cardiovascular fitness. Its six branches are progressive and linked. You should always start your Heart Zone Training program with your current level of conditioning in mind. Novices should begin on the first or "base" branch, then slowly climb each of the six branches to the tree top. If you are a conditioned athlete, you can start further up the tree. The training tree allows you to add different components to your training as you become more fit. This is exactly how Olympic athletes train, but it's also how beginners should train, climbing to one branch at a time in order to build muscle strength and obtain aerobic conditioning.

Step 5: Set Your Weekly Training Time

Be realistic about time. Most of us never have enough time to do everything we should or want to do. Think of time as a checking account. Each day you get a twenty-four-hour deposit, and though you spend it all by day's end, sometimes it seems you've accomplished little. Unfortunately, we often sacrifice our workouts first. Insist that exercise be one of the most essential and important parts of your day. I have found it best to set up a weekly workout schedule and commit myself to it.

Step 6: Calculate Your Time-In-Zone (TIZ)

When you heart zone train, you need to apply your valuable exercise minutes within the zones that match your goals. TIZ is calculated as a percentage of your total training time. Your limb on the training tree indicates how much time you should spend in-zone. You can do multiple or double zone workouts or distribute your time in other ways. If you are just beginning, you'll spend 100 percent of your time on the Base limb, working out almost exclusively in Z1, the Healthy Heart zone. Stay between the floor and ceiling of Z1 for four to six weeks before you climb up to the next limb, Endurance.

Step 7: Determine Your Weekly HZT Points

Keeping track of your exercise points provides both motivation and rewards. One minute equals one point in Z1, and each time you move up one zone you multiply the effect of your exercise. Working out in Z3, for example, equals three times the points of working in Z1.

Start by determining how many Heart Zone Training points your workout plan will earn you. Then pause to consider whether you're being realistic. Ask yourself, "Will this plan really work for me?" As the weeks go by, add points by training longer or working out in progressively higher zones. The more points you earn, the more total calories you expend. Establish a modest initial goal, such as 150 points a week. Get comfortable at that total for several weeks or a few months before you move gradually to 200 points, then to 350 points, then to 500 points. Try to add twenty-five to fifty points after several weeks. Once you become truly fit, you might even reward yourself with 1,000 points, as I do.

Step 8: Do Your Workouts

Doing my planned Heart Zone Training workouts is my number-one favorite part of the day. Planning is essential to success in any endeavor, but nothing matches the exhilaration of executing that plan.

When you get comfortable with exercising regularly, you'll love this step too, because movement designed by and for you gives you the greatest "buzz" of all. I call it "the glow," and it's high energy.

Prepare yourself for interruptions to your plan. It happens to all of us. If you miss a workout, let it go. You don't need to do a double workout the next day. However, do take time to evaluate the obstacles that disrupted your training and reset your schedule as needed to minimize interruptions in the future.

Step 9: Fill in Your HZT Points Log

Maintaining any sort of log, whether a diary, a record of your fat intake and caloric output, or your appointment schedule, rewards you by giving you a concrete picture of your accomplishments. You can look back and review both your successes and your failures, and you can compare one week with another. I love to keep logs, not only because they tell me what I've done but because they help me plan what I should do next. By keeping a careful log, I discovered that something always happens—an injury, a respiratory infection, staleness—when my training reaches 2,000 points a week. Now I rarely earn that many points because I know that by doing so I will risk the setbacks that arise from overtraining.

Step 10: Complete Monthly Self-Tests

Along the Heart Zone Training journey you should periodically measure improvement by self-testing. I self-test with a 1-mile walk, a 1-mile run, or a 3-mile bike ride, using my Z3 mid-point heart rate as a steady gauge. To test your improvement, you might use your Z2 or Z3 mid-point heart rate as your own gauge. After a warm-up, reach your mid-point and hold steady at that heart rate for the duration of the test. As you become fitter, the elapsed time for the test will shorten. When you lose fitness, the test will take longer at the same heart rate. Another useful self-test involves checking your resting heart rate on a regular basis. Your resting heart rate should always remain within a five-beat window. If it rises above that range, then you should possibly make a change in your workout that day: Your body is sending a strong biofeedback message that something is stressing you physically. Your body responds to that stress by raising your resting heart rate.

The Heart Zone Training Chart

To help you put all ten steps to Heart Zone Training together, here is a chart that shows heart rate zones based on maximum heart rate. Photocopy this chart and use it. It's a nice, concise way of looking at most of the information in this book on one page. Find your maximum heart rate in the top row, then look below it to see the heart rate range for each zone.

HEART ZONE TRAINING CHART

ZONE NUMBER	ZONE NAME	150 BPM	155 BPM	160 BPM	165 BPM	170 BPM	175 BPM	180 BPM	185 BPM	190 BPM	195 BPM	200 BPM	205 BPM	210 BPM	215 BPM	220 BPM
Z5	Redline 90%–100%	135–150	140–155	144–160	149–165	153–170	158–175	162–180	167–185	171–190	176–195	180–200	185–205	189–210	194–215	198–220
Z4	Threshold 80%–90%	120–135	124–140	128–144	132–149	136–153	140–158	144–162	148–167	152–171	156–146	160–180	164–185	168–189	172–194	176–198
Z3	Aerobic 70%–80%	105–120	109–124	112–128	116–132	119–136	123–140	126–144	130–148	133–152	137–156	140–160	144–164	147–168	151–172	154–176
Z2	Temperate 60%–70%	90–105	93–109	96–112	99–116	102–119	105–123	108–126	111–130	114–133	117–137	120–140	123–144	126–147	129–151	132–154
Z1	Healthy Heart 50%–60%	75–90	78–93	80–96	83–99	85–102	88–105	90–108	93–111	95–114	98–117	100–120	103–123	105–126	108–129	110–132

Keeping Fit Without Ever Losing "Heart"

Believe it or not, every once in a while, I toss my Heart Zone Training program to the wind and train solo without my heart rate monitor. While you want to make Heart Zone Training a weekly habit, you don't want it to become an addiction. I often end up chuckling at myself for thinking I base my training on strict science, when I know that perceived effort and other subjective feelings also figure in my training. Occasionally I run free for a while, just getting high on my speed and distance; but when I strap that monitor watch back on my wrist and try to guess my intensity level, I usually discover that I've been thinking I'm working harder than my heart rate actually indicates. After more than fifteen years of training by heart rate and seeing all that it has brought me in athletic improvement and success, I still find hard information more powerful than guessing.

Maintain a goal of optimum all-around fitness, but remain flexible as your body changes, as your performances change, and as your time available for exercising changes. The best goal remains the same whether you are an Olympic champion or a septuagenarian athlete. That goal is to become as fit as possible, given all the changes that will occur in your life.

Whatever your age, gender, or present level of fitness, it takes a lot of heart (blood-plumping capacity) and a lot of "heart" (confidence and inspiration) to achieve your best-possible performance. Measuring your heart rate with or without a monitor can help you build both your muscled heart and your feeling heart.

Building your "pumping heart" is the principal goal of your Heart Zone Training program. That program, monitored carefully, builds your heart's pumping efficiency. Little information has been offered by experts about using your monitor to build the "inspired" heart, though all the experts agree that peak athletic performance is 50 percent perspiration and 50 percent inspiration. How do you develop both? I want to give you some parting advice about using your heart rate monitor to bring forth the sort of inspired heart that leads to highest exercise and training fulfillment.

I encourage you to match your training heart with your inspired heart. Delve into that feeling of the pumping heart and the body's resultant energy expenditure. At what heart rate pace do you find your mind and body flowing along effortlessly? How do you feel? What does your breathing sound like? What muscles are working the hardest, and how does their working affect your technique? Explore your pumping heart and feeling heart simultaneously. Olympic athletes do this all the time, searching for new discoveries about themselves, and so should you. Tune in to how you feel both physically and mentally at various heart rates so that you can begin to develop the sixth sense—the two hearts fusing into one. Over time you'll learn that you can easily flow into this state of fusion at will.

This sixth sense can also help you deal effectively with what ultimately happens to all of us with the passage of time as we continue to heart zone train. Any fitness program should take into account the aging process. My friend Paul, now seventy-five years old, has trained with me for more than twenty years. Having Heart Zone Trained exclusively for the past three years, he called the other day for a little advice and support. He has, he confided, begun to slow down and doesn't know whether he can maintain his 165 bpm marathon heart rate pace and still run under nine minutes per mile for the 26.2-mile marathon distance next month. I challenged him to try, because I know him well enough to think his "inspired" heart will lead him to the finish line.

Given the inevitable and sometimes uncomfortable effects of aging on the body, exercise and training become even more important. The Heart Zone Training program offers unique individuals not only a universal application to all sports and fitness activities but also a lifetime of benefit. Use it to monitor and manage your own body's aging process.

Think for a minute about some of the people you have met in this book. Remember Amy, who yo-yo exercised for years until she discovered the Z2 Healthy Heart zone and found success? Recall my brother Chris, an avid runner, who was forced to slow down into the Healthy Heart zone in order to lower his high blood pressure successfully? Margaret, my colleague, recovering from a minor heart attack, who got back on track with her first exercise program? And how about Brad, who worked out at lunch to lose that extra fat? When each of them began Heart Zone Training, they launched themselves on a course that would help them achieve their very different goals. Then there was my next-door neighbor, Christine, who suffered from "chronic exercise aversion" to exercise and wasted money on membership dues at the club she never visited. She now loves working out on the machines using Heart Zone Training, as does Michael, who keeps laughing his way to fitness.

All of these success stories remind me of my office mate, Ellen, a forty-five-year-old marathon runner. Heart Zone Training has changed her life more than anyone I know.

When we met several years ago, Ellen was taking heavy-duty medication for high blood pressure, had gained fifteen pounds in five years, and was unhappy in her work. Her father had died of a heart attack at the age of forty-one, and she worried about following him to an early grave. To her credit, however, Ellen did not sink into depression; instead, she seized the opportunity to take a hard look at her life and make some tough choices. For her, that meant walking away from a secure but high-stress job and living frugally in order to launch a new business doing what she loves—writing and motivating others to make healthy lifestyle choices.

At about 11:00 one morning, two months after her career shift, Ellen appeared in the office with a big jug of orange juice and a mini bottle of champagne. As she filled two glasses, she announced, "We have a big event to celebrate." I couldn't help but wonder why we were drinking even a small amount of alcohol at 11:00 in the morning, but I figured she had a good reason, so I hoisted my glass to hers. "Here's my toast," she said. "My blood pressure has dropped to normal and soon I will be off medication." She had accomplished this amazing goal by putting all the components of her life together with Heart Zone Training. Unlike her father, who suffered silently with coronary heart disease and high blood pressure, Ellen took her health and her lifestyle into control, using Heart Zone Training for every workout.

Like Ed Oswalt and every other heart zone trainer, Ellen faithfully followed the Ten Steps of Heart Zone Training to accomplish her highest and inner-most goals. I have seen it work again and again, and I know in my heart of hearts that it will work for you. All you need to do is eat a low-fat, balanced diet, exercise in the heart zones, set small goals and accomplish them one at a time, and, above all, manage your health by monitoring and measuring it. Design a personal program. Plan and log your workouts. Take control of your own health. Share your experience with others, and encourage them to get started on their own creative programs. Write to me—2636 Fulton Avenue, Sacramento, CA 95821—with any questions or thoughts about Heart Zone Training. I'll answer your questions and share your success with others.

This is the end of the book, but it marks the beginning of a new health and wellness and fitness revolution. Having read it and taken its advice to heart, you have put yourself on the leading edge of that revolution, a whole new way of looking at fitness based on personalization and creativity and design.

It all starts by identifying what you love and filling your life with it. I love that feeling of being alive and possessing the confidence that I can do whatever I set out to accomplish. The heart is an incredible muscle, and different from every other organ in the body. It's the true link between the mind and the body and between the body and the soul. Love your hearts, both the pump and the inspiration, and take good care of them both because the way to your soul is through your heart.

The Beginning

Appendix
Choosing a Heart Rate Monitor

By Ellen E. Sampson, Editor
The Fitness Monitor, the heart rate monitor newsletter

Just a decade ago, heart rate monitors were used by only a handful of top athletes. Thanks to technological advances and market forces, monitors are now affordable and available to athletes and fitness enthusiasts of every caliber. Making the decision to buy a monitor is relatively easy, but picking one to fit your needs and budget requires careful consideration. Here are a few hints to help in your decision making.

First and foremost, do not confuse a heart rate monitor with a pulse meter. They are not the same. A heart rate monitor records your heart's electrical impulses and gives accurate readings of your heart rate. Pulse meters, on the other hand, detect the heart rate signal by emitting a light wave that passes through the blood vessels (usually in your finger tip or ear lobe) and is interrupted by the pulse wave occurring with each heart contraction. This older technology is very sensitive to changes in light and is simply not reliable or accurate enough for Heart Zone Training. Buy a heart rate monitor, not a pulse meter.

Also, don't be confused by the terms "heart rate monitor" and "heart rate watch." Both are heart rate monitors, but heart rate watches also have typical watch functions such as time of day and date which ordinary monitors do not.

Wireless heart rate monitors generally consist of three components: a wrist receiver, which receives the heart rate signal; a chest strap; and a chest transmitter, which transmits a heart rate signal to the receiver. Depending upon the brand, the transmitter may snap onto the front of a chest strap with built-in electrodes, or it may be a one-piece unit with enclosed electrodes.

Both the transmitter and receiver require batteries that will eventually need to be replaced. Some units are designed for simple do-it-yourself battery replacement, while others must be handled by authorized representatives, or the warranty will be invalidated.

The terms "functions" or "features" refer to the different capabilities of particular monitors. There are currently more than two dozen different models of wireless monitors on the market; collectively they offer numerous features. Depending upon your goals and budget, you may need or want a monitor with multiple functions.

The Basic Monitor

Continuous-read heart rate monitors are the most basic kind of monitors. They do one thing and one thing only—display your heart rate, usually in large digital numbers. A continuous-read monitor is among the least-expensive wireless model available and can be purchased for less than $100. This model is also the easiest to use: Just strap it on.

Added Functions to Consider

Although some monitor manufacturers have introduced specialized features unique to their own models, most brands offer many universal functions. The names of these functions may vary, so be sure you understand what they do.

Monitors with **watch functions**, such as time of day and date, are especially popular, because they eliminate the need to wear both a monitor and watch. Several brands give the option of using a twelve- or a twenty-four-hour clock. Many models with a watch function split the display screen and show time and heart rate simultaneously. A monitor with watch functions may or may not have all the capabilities of a sports watch.

Another popular feature, **programmable hi-low heart rate zones**, allows you to set a specific workout zone. If your heart rate exceeds or drops below the set zone, an audio alarm will usually sound, or you may see a visual indicator such as an arrow or blinking number. Some monitors allow you to program any zone, such as 143 to 152 bpm. Other monitors limit hi-low functions to five-beat increments such as 140 to 150 bpm or 145-155 bpm. If you work out with others, consider buying a monitor that allows you to turn off the audio alarm. The beeping can become annoying to friends who don't share your enthusiasm for Heart Zone Training.

Memory or recall functions are useful to monitor users who want to do more than watch their heart rates during workouts. Memory functions allow you to recall certain heart readings after your workout is over. These readings will vary according to your specific monitor brand and model.

One common recall function will tell you how much time you spend **in, over, and below** your designated zone. Several upper-end models will also indicate your **average heart rate**. Some models allow you to specify the time **intervals** to record, such as thirty seconds. At the end of the workout you can then recall your recording and see what your heart rate was every thirty seconds.

Monitors with **stopwatch and lap features** function much like a combination sports watch and heart rate monitor with recall. By hitting your lap button at any interval, for example, you can go back later and see both time and the corresponding heart rate. This feature is similar to the interval recall function, except the interval is not pre-determined.

Frequently, a monitor with stopwatch features also includes one or more **pace-interval alarms**. This should not be confused with the daily alarms or hi-low alarms found on some monitors. The pace-interval alarm sounds on a time interval that you program into the monitor.

One word of caution about alarms in general: Some are louder than others. Most alarms, however, are hard to discern in noisy environments such as gyms and busy roads.

Specialized Features

Most but not all monitors are **water-resistant** and can be used during swimming or in inclement weather. If you know this feature is essential for your needs, review the warranty and use instructions carefully. Do not, under any circumstances, press monitor buttons under the water. This could allow water into the unit and reduce its life.

Many manufacturers also offer **special mounts** that allow you to attach your monitor to bicycles or other kinds of fitness equipment. These mounts are sometimes included with a monitor at no additional cost or may be available for a separate add-on price.

The **computer-related accessories and capabilities** of monitors are just now beginning to broaden. Using a computer interface unit and software, you can download recorded heart rate data for analysis and graphic display. One available model even allows you to watch your heart rate on your computer screen while you work out indoors. There are also computer programs on the market that enable you to incorporate heart zone records in your computerized training log.

Whatever monitor features you seek, be a conscientious consumer by studying available options and comparing prices of similar units. The monitor market is changing rapidly, and retailers and manufacturers are always discounting older models as more sophisticated units become available. Be sure you are getting the features you need and want. If you're sincere about Heart Zone Training, select a model with the most features you can afford. Many users end up buying a second monitor during their first year because they find they want additional capabilities.

Finally, keep in mind that all the features and functions on the market won't make your Heart Zone Training effective unless you learn to use your monitor. After buying a monitor, take the time to read the instruction manual from cover to cover at least once and spend an hour fooling around with the buttons until you can program it easily.

The Fitness Monitor, a four- to eight-page newsletter for heart rate monitor users, is published bi-monthly. U.S. subscriptions are $24/year. For a sample or more information, write, 2636 Fulton Avenue, Sacramento, CA 95821; or call 916/451-7043 (phone/fax).

Glossary of Terms

Aerobic: Technically, *aerobic* means "in the presence of oxygen"; *aerobic* metabolism utilizes oxygen. In everyday use the term means exercising at an *intensity* level at which you can still breathe comfortably and talk conversationally.

Ambient Heart Rate: The number of times per minute that your heart contracts when you are sedentary, sitting and relaxed.

Anaerobic: Technically, *anaerobic* means "in the absence of oxygen." During *anaerobic* metabolism the burning of calories does not involve oxygen. In everyday use the term means exercising at an intensity level when your body goes into an overload state and where you can only continue to exercise for a limited period.

Anaerobic Threshold: Also commonly known as the "lactate threshold," this is the heart rate point at which *lactic acid* produced in the muscle tissue begins to accumulate at a faster rate in the blood stream than the body can utilize it. This point is the ceiling or the uppermost limit a body can sustain aerobically.

Cardiac: Having to do with the heart muscle.

Cardiac Output: The volume of blood pumped from the heart each minute, calculated by multiplying the heart rate by the volume from each stroke, or heart contraction.

Cool-Down: That period after exercise when you slowly allow yourself to return to your *ambient heart rate* and your body temperature moves down toward normal. Also known as "warm-down."

Dehydration: Loss of essential body fluids, especially water.

Deconditioned: Out of shape, untrained, at a low level of fitness.

Duration: The length of time you exercise or the distance you travel, sometimes measured in terms of calories burned.

Electrocardiogram (ECG): A print-out or graphic recording of electrical activity during the heart muscle's contractions.

Endurance: The ability to exercise over long periods of time without getting unduly tired.

Fartlek: A Swedish term for "speed play," which means varying the speed of the exercise intermittently and playfully. An example would be running hard between every other telephone pole.

Fat: A food substance that the body converts into an energy source and that it can easily store for future use.

Fitness: A varying condition of physical well-being, combining *aerobic* ability, muscle strength, and flexibility.

Frequency: The number of workouts you perform per day or per week.

Glucose: An energy source transported in the bloodstream that comes mostly from ingested sugar.

Glycogen: The stored form of *glucose*, usually found in the liver and muscles.

Heart Rate: The number or frequency of contractions, which can be inferred from *pulse* rate (expansion of the artery resulting from the beat of the heart).

Heart Rate Monitor: A wrist watch-like device that measures the electrical activity of the heart in beats per minute.

Intensity: The level of exertion or degree of effort.

Interval Training: A training technique that alternates between short, intense efforts of exercise and periods of rest.

Lactic Acid: A chemical in the blood that accumulates as a result of high-intensity exercise. High levels of *lactic acid* in the bloodstream reduce the body's ability to contract specific muscles and inhibit fat metabolism and enzyme activity.

Maximum Oxygen Uptake: A measurement of the amount of oxygen that the body can consume at a given time. Experts consider *maximum oxygen uptake* the "gold standard" test of aerobic fitness. A high *maximum oxygen uptake,* also known as VO_2 Max, or consumption, means a higher level of fitness conditioning.

Myocardium: The heart muscle.

Nutrition: The ingestion of adequate energy or calories, including a balance of fat, carbohydrates, protein, vitamins, minerals, and water.

Obesity: Having too much body fat; commonly defined as 30 percent body fat or more for women and 20 percent body fat or more for men.

Overload: A greater amount of exercise *intensity* or workload than the body part can comfortably handle.

Overtraining: Exercising in excess or beyond what is healthy. It raises the risk of staleness, illness, or injury.

Oxygen Debt: An accumulated deficit of the oxygen required for metabolism to replace what has been used up during exercise.

Glossary of Terms

Perceived Exertion: A subjective estimate of exercise *intensity* measured by a scale known as the RPE, or rating of perceived exertion.

Power: The application of strength and speed; the rate of exercise measured by multiplying force by velocity.

Pulse: The blood flow wave that travels down the artery after each contraction of the heart, used to measure *heart rate*. Pulse rate measures the biomechanical flow of blood from each heart beat.

Resistance Training: Lifting weights, or any kind of training in which muscle strength is enhanced.

Risk Factors: Events or behaviors associated with a higher potential for developing disease. Coronary *risk factors* increase the risk of heart disease.

Stroke Volume: The amount or volume of blood pumped from the *ventricle* during each contraction of the heart.

Threshold: The minimum activity required to elicit a specific response.

Training Zone: A heart rate zone or range of heart beats used during exercise. Different training effects occur as the result of time spent exercising within a *training zone.*

Ventricle: The chamber of the heart that pumps blood to the lung on the right side or to the rest of the body on the left side.

Warm-Up: The activity before you begin your main exercise program, used to increase muscle temperature and range of motion.

Workload: Force expressed through distance in a certain amount of time, or frequency multiplied by time.

Zone Training: A method of training based on using *heart rate intensity* to produce a desired exercise effect.

Index

Index